Sun Proof

A Practical Guide for Sun-Damaged Skin

How-To Maximize Prevention

and Repair the Damage

By Austin Cope, MD, MBA

Disclaimer

The information provided in this book is designed to provide helpful information on the subjects discussed. This book is not meant to be used, nor should it be used, to diagnose or treat any medical condition. For diagnosis or treatment of any medical problem, consult your own physician. The publisher and author are not responsible for any specific health or dermatology needs that may require medical supervision and are not liable for any damages or negative consequences from any treatment, action, application or preparation, to any person reading or following the information in this book. References are provided for informational purposes only and do not constitute endorsement of any websites or other sources. Readers should be aware that the websites, products, brand names, and others listed in this book may change.

For more information and additional content please visit
Sunproofbook.com

Testimonials

"I recently had a procedure performed by Dr. Cope and WOW, he is awesome! I greatly appreciate his positive attitude, friendliness, patience, skill, and knowledge. He took his time to explain what to expect before and after the procedure--and my result was OUTSTANDING! Dr. Cope clearly is passionate about his work and is exceptionally people oriented. I'm looking forward to seeing him in the future!"

-Sheri B.

"Dr. Cope was very knowledgeable and took his time with me choosing which injectable was best fit. He is an awesome doctor, injector, and all around great person. Highly recommend seeing him for all of your needs."

-Fontes C.

"I went in to see Dr Cope to have filler put in my lips & he recommended some other treatments that would benefit me more to start with. He has created a step by step plan to create a more youthful appearance to my skin. I'm so excited to see the end result!!! He takes his time & explains everything. I felt very comfortable. I would highly recommend him. He knows his stuff."

-Lisa L.

"I had been having awful TMJ pain and repeated tension headaches. I went and saw Dr. Cope and he was able to use Botox to treat my TMJ. The relief I have felt has been amazing! The pain has gone away and I am no longer clenching my jaw. I would highly recommend this treatment. Dr. Cope is a great advocate and a very friendly, kind person. You can't find a better doctor!"

-Amy G.

Table of Contents

Before and After Photos

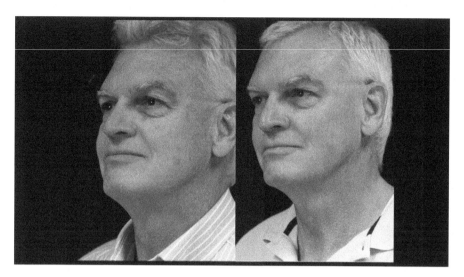

Photo by Austin Cope, MD, MBA

Before(L)/After(R) of patient with moderate sun damage. Treatments included: Aggressive topical therapy for discoloration, chemotherapy cream for pre-cancers, and 2 rounds of Fotona Micropeel "Goldilocks" laser for improving skin tone and texture. (Chapters 4, 7, 8)

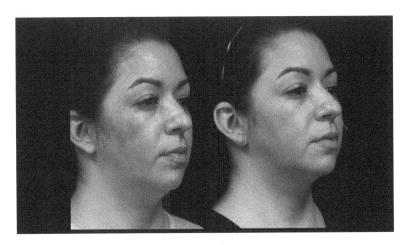

Photo by Austin Cope, MD, MBA

Before(L)/After(R) of patient with previously unresponsive melasma present for years. Current treatments that finally worked: Aggressive topical therapy x3 months and two rounds of medium-depth chemical peels. (Chapters 3, 7)

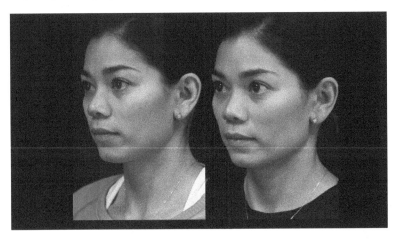

Photo by Austin Cope, MD, MBA

Before(L)/After(R) of patient with new-onset sun spots (solar lentigo) on the left cheek. Treatments included strong topical therapy combined with repeat gentle laser procedures (Clear and Brilliant). (Chapters 3, 4, 7)

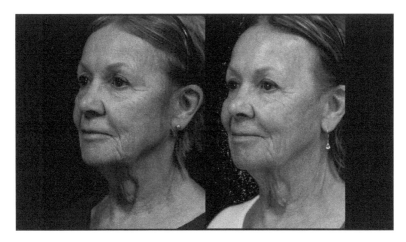

Photo by Austin Cope, MD, MBA

Before(L)/After(R) of patient with severe sun damage. She was treated with ultra-strong laser (fully-ablative) and had a fantastic result. Downtime was significant, but she feels it was definitely worth it and she is very happy with the results. (Chapter 4)

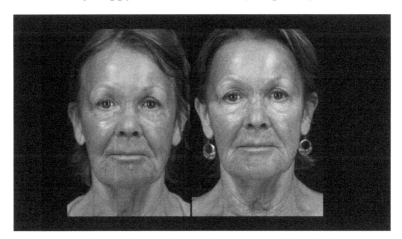

Photo by Austin Cope, MD, MBA

Healing photos of the previous patient who had a recent fully-ablative laser procedure. Day 2 (L) and Day 4 (R) respectively. One week of true downtime with complete sun avoidance is critical for these procedures. (Chapter 4)

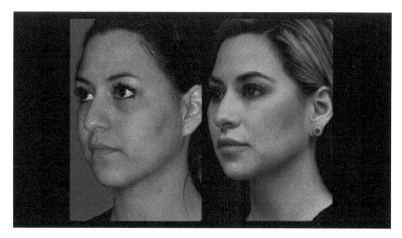

Photo By Jody Comstock, MD

Before(L)/After(R) of a patient after dermal filler injections. Areas treated include the cheeks, jawline, and lips. She says she feels more confident and more like her true self.

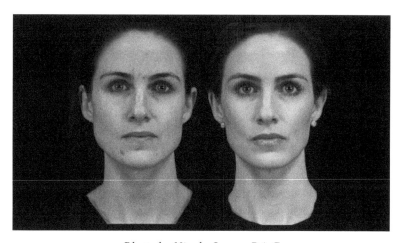

Photo by Nicole James, PA-C

Before(L)/After(R) of a patient with acne and masseter hypertrophy (jawline muscle). Treatment of the acne included aggressive topical therapy and some light lasers to target the redness. Treatment of the jawline was one session of Botox injections. She is very happy with these results, especially the narrower jawline.

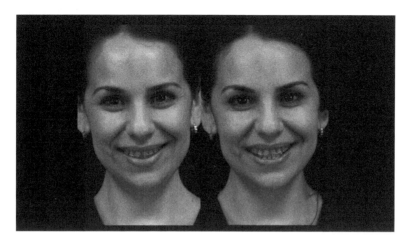

Before(L)/After(R) of a patient after Botox injections of the lateral eye area (crows feet). In the right photo she is trying to squint to activate this area, but is unable to recreate the crows feet. She is very happy with these results and says this makes her feel more confident about herself.

Introduction

If you live on the planet earth, then you've likely noticed how your skin ages with time. And rightfully so. Your skin puts up with a lot. It gets cuts and bruises every time you fall. It gets punctured and scratched from your dog. It gets submerged underwater for long periods of time when you bathe or go swimming. It fights off foreign invaders and gets exposed to poison ivy. And above all, it protects you from a daily onslaught of the biggest villain of all--ultraviolet light! It does all this to try to keep your insides safe and to keep you alive.

Your skin also gives you your unique "look" and personality. You wouldn't be you without that skin on your face. It's the first thing you see in the morning and the last thing you see at night. And yes, you've noticed that it changes over time. It ages and looks different. Just look at a picture from your wedding day or high school graduation. What's different? Likely a lot. And it can be hard to put your finger on it. Your brain recognizes the differences in a nanosecond, but you have a hard time localizing and quantifying the changes.

Unfortunately, as your skin starts to sag, so does your confidence. You feel like you're losing an important part of yourself. You still feel young and energetic; shouldn't your outward appearance still show that? The answer is a resounding YES!

You can still look as young as you feel. You can defy the aging process and look 5, 10, or even 20 years younger than your chronological age. But it takes work. It's like the bodybuilder or marathon runner who has put in years of consistent work to achieve amazing results. You can do the same with your skin.

It all hinges on how you protect yourself from the sun. That's right, the sun is the villain in this story. I know that it produces light for us to see, warmth so we can survive, and it gives life to our entire planet. But for our purposes in considering photodamage, it is the villain. But it's a villain that we can't get away from, so we need to learn to live with it. And even, perhaps, enjoy it without letting it damage our DNA and break down our collagen. Yes, this can be done. Let me show you how.

Chapter 1

Sun Damage

Incredible Organ

Most people don't think of the skin as an organ, just a covering that you want to keep looking nice. The truth is that the skin is an incredible living organ, just like your heart, kidneys, lungs, liver, intestines, eyes, and others. The skin has so many jobs that it is difficult to name them all in one sitting. But here's an incomplete list to give us some insights. (V = function that is vital to life, and if this function is lost then life is emergently threatened.)

- Skin gives you your personalized "look."
- Skin forms a protective barrier to keep things out (V).
- Skin attacks and kills invaders that attempt to get in (V).
- Skin protects from sun damage (V).
- Skin thermoregulates to keep the body at a proper temperature (V).
- Skin allows for movement of underlying muscles and joints without tearing or breaking (V).
- Skin forms proper cushioning and support for internal organs.
- Your sense of touch is an intricate and amazing "joint venture" between the nervous system and the skin (V).

All these functions happen day-to-day, minute-to-minute, and mostly without being recognized or appreciated. But the skin moves on, performing its vital functions that keep us safe, protected, and alive.

As the World Turns and the Skin Ages

What's interesting about the skin is that it's the organ you see every day. You look in the mirror and see your skin. You don't see your heart, lungs, kidneys, liver, bones, or muscles. For this reason, you may care disproportionately more about your skin than the "invisible organs" of your body. You notice when there's a new spot, a new blemish, or something doesn't look quite like it used to. In short, you notice the natural aging process of your skin. You may even notice that some parts of your skin are aging faster than others. You may notice, for example, that the skin on your right forearm looks different from the skin on your right hip. Or wondered, "Why is the skin on my older sibling looking better and younger than mine?" There are many components that lead to aging skin, but by far the biggest is sun exposure. Your hips and your forearms have had dramatically different amounts of sun exposure over the years. You and your siblings may have had similar amounts of sun exposure growing up, but that all changed as you became adults and led different lives. I have seen 80-year-olds who look like they're 60, and 30-year-olds who look like they're 50. Of course, genetics plays a role, and not all skin types are the same. But of this you can be sure: The amount of aging on your skin is directly influenced by the amount of sun exposure you have had (and continue to have).

Tucson, We Have a Problem

I have a great little family consisting of my wife, five kids, and myself. We moved around a lot during my medical training and thought we could handle just about any new place. Then we made the mistake of moving to Tucson, Arizona, in the middle of June. I could not believe that any place on the planet could be so hot (and I grew up in the Mojave Desert of Southern Utah)! We almost didn't survive when our air conditioner went out that first week. However, we recovered and got used to this "new normal." We quickly fell in love with Tucson and the unique and natural beauty. Now one of our favorite things to do is watch the magical sunsets behind the beautiful silhouetted saguaro cacti. At a certain point of the evening the sky just seems to glow, which to me is some form of magic. Tucson has so many wonderful things to offer. Most of them include going outside. It's a veritable outdoor wonderland. I couldn't believe my first winter when I didn't have to get my "winter bin" out of storage. I think I wore a T-shirt the entire winter just to prove to myself that I could. This is presumably why so many people flock to Arizona during the winter months. The downside is that we have a lot more opportunities to harm our skin.

Arizona ranks highest for the number of sunny days in the entire country. As dermatologists, this explains why we see so much sun damage and so many skin cancers. Everyone in Arizona is at risk for these problems. By spending time in Arizona, your skin is high- risk. Sunlight damages skin. Every time. Constantly. Cumulatively. A great corollary to this is smoking. We all know that smoking is terrible. Smoking causes cancer. It ruins lives. And most of us have developed a deep opposition to smoking. Sun exposure is in the same category. It damages, it harms, and it destroys. But the big difference here is that we can't escape it. The sun surrounds us every day. Many of us (rightfully so) are actively seeking outdoor activities that are bathed in it. We, as a society, have not developed the same opposition to sun exposure that we have to smoking. And here's the bottom line: If you do nothing about your regular sun exposure, then you will develop terrible skin--diseased, damaged, discolored, and cancerous.

Sneaky Sun Exposure

If you're reading this book, then you are probably already aware of the dangers of sun exposure. When you go outside for prolonged periods of time (hiking, biking, gardening, swimming, beach, and so on) you probably cover up in sunscreen or protective clothing. Good for you. That's a big win. You're doing better than millions of people who are still sunbathing and going to tanning beds. Some of you may be thinking, "But I hardly ever go outside." I get this comment all the time when discussing sun damage with my patients. Most of them don't realize how much time they actually spend in the sun, so they never put on sunscreen. There are sneaky categories of sun exposure that just about everyone is getting every day. These are enough to cause considerable damage in and of themselves, even if you're not outside gardening, hiking, swimming, or walking. They are cumulative and they add up. They are the biggest reason you look older every year. The following are a few examples of sneaky sun exposure that you may not have considered.

Parking Lot Sun

Chances are that you run various errands throughout the day. You probably go to lunch, meet friends, visit family, go to the gym, go grocery shopping, go to the library, mail a package, or do any number of other tasks. The average person spends about ten minutes of their day walking to and from their car, often in a large parking lot. This is direct sun exposure that you likely haven't accounted for. If you are like the average person, then you are getting about 70 minutes of direct, unprotected sun exposure every week. What would happen to your skin if you went outside in direct sunlight for 70 continuous minutes? You would get a sunburn. The damage would be obvious. But since it occurs throughout the week, it's not obvious. It's silent and imperceptible, but it is damaging your skin all the same.

Windows (UVA and UVB)

You may have heard that the windows in your car and house block 99% of sunlight. This, for the most part, is false. There are two important types of ultraviolet light: UVA and UVB. UVB is higher energy and shorter wavelength and causes more superficial damage to the skin. It's a big player in most skin cancers. UVB is blocked by most windows. UVA, however, is lower energy and longer wavelength. It goes through windows and through the most superficial layers of skin. UVA causes deeper damage to the skin, which leads to more of the textural changes. This leads to thin and wrinkly skin that we associate with aging. Many sunscreens do not cover UVA. In fact, in the US we have no systematic way of measuring how well this gets blocked. SPF is strictly a marker of UVB blockage.

I often see patients who have significantly more damage on their left side than their right. I'll ask them if they know why that is. Less than half of them know the answer--driver's side sun. When you drive you get significantly more sun damage (UVA) on the left side of your body. If you have more damage on your right side, then you either live in the UK, or you're more often a passenger than a driver. There are some fascinating photos online of long-term truck drivers. The left side of their faces often looks 10 or 20 years older than the right side.

Visible Light and Infrared Light

Few people know that visible light, infrared light, and pollution also cause significant damage to the skin. The damage may not be as dramatic as the UV spectra, but these things are everywhere, including indoors. Even the screens from our devices (which are frequently right next to our faces) emit significant amounts of these types of light. These can even cause flareups in certain skin conditions like lupus or melasma. They also contribute to brown spots and dyspigmentation in the skin.

Skin Pigment and Latitude

It's no mystery that there are a variety of skin types with varying amounts of natural pigment produced. Ethnic groups with ancestors living nearer to the equator have developed skin with darker pigment. And ethnic groups living nearer the poles of the earth have developed lighter skin types with less pigment. This was simply an evolutionary adaptation based on the amount of UV damage each ethnic group received over time. What we can learn from this is fascinating. Near the equator, with higher levels of direct sunlight, there is a SURVIVAL ADVANTAGE to having more UV protection. This makes intuitive sense. But the problem we're faced with now is that many of us are ill-suited for our current environments. Our ancestors lived in places dramatically different from those we are now living in. This means our skin adapts poorly to the amount of UV damage we are receiving. This is the case for most people of European descent living in America.

If you fall into this category, then your skin is likely to be poorly adapted to your current environment. The latitude range of the US is about 30-40° N, while the latitude range of Northern Europe is about 50-65° N. This difference is dramatic. To illustrate further, the latitude of

Arizona is identical to that of Afghanistan (33° N). Clearly, the fair skin of most people living in Phoenix is not well suited for life in Phoenix or Afghanistan. The native groups of the Mediterranean, Middle East, Northern Africa, and Southern Asia all have skin types that are better equipped for this level of damaging sun exposure. Northern Europeans have adapted to far less direct sunlight during long winters of excessive darkness, significant cloud coverage, and mild/short summers. In many ways, the world we live in has been turned upside down by relatively recent migration and travel patterns. This is an important and foundational concept to understand. It's why you are at such high risk every time you walk outside.

Wait, The Sun Causes Wrinkles?

I remember as a kid laying out in my yard, at the pool, or at the beach. I loved the nice little tan I would get and wanted to make sure every possible inch of my skin could have some. You probably know what I'm talking about: laying out covered in baby oil and maybe with a reflection mirror for good measure. My father was a physician and told me, "If you get too much sun you might get skin cancer when you're older." I performed a quick cost/benefit analysis in my head.

If I get a nice tan as a teenager.

- **Cost**: I might get skin cancer when I'm old.
- **Benefit**: My skin will look great now.

Guess which argument won? That's right, getting a tan won every time.

Here was my reasoning.

1. I want to look great to get noticed by girls.
2. I like the way my skin looks when it's tan, and presumably, the girls do, too.

3. I don't care if I get skin cancer when I'm old--I'll be old, and that's a million years away.
4. Getting skin cancer is not a guarantee; it's a MAYBE.
5. Plus, my dad's a doctor and can help me recognize and remove any skin cancer I may get.
6. Also, don't they say we need to get a lot of sun for vitamin D?

I felt that my justification for continuing to tan was great: big short-term benefit with mild and mitigated long term risk. Plus, I was even doing my body good with this whole vitamin D thing (more on this later).

Boy was I wrong. I overplayed the benefit of tanning and vitamin D, underplayed the true cost of skin cancer, and completely left out one of the most important arguments--wrinkles! That's right, wrinkles! The sun causes wrinkles! And they don't wait until you're old; they happen now. For some skin types they can happen in your 20s! And they're directly caused by sun exposure. So my original cost/benefit analysis should have looked like this.

If I get a tan in my teens/20s:

- **Cost**: I will have thin, wrinkled, blotchy skin for the rest of my life, starting in my 20s and 30s. I will consistently look like the oldest person in the room.
- **Benefit**: Wait, what was the benefit again?

Daily Habits

As you read this book, hopefully you will see how real and scary sun damage can be. Hopefully, you will also see how this damage can be prevented and reduced. You can still live a full and fun outdoor life, even in Arizona. It all comes down to prevention and daily habits. Either you will have bad sun habits or good sun habits. And the delta between those two things grows and grows until there's a dramatic and visible difference. Brian Tracy, motivational public speaker and self-development author says, "Successful people are simply those with successful habits." It is my hope that you will pick up or solidify a successful sun habit or two from this book. And if you already have sun damage, don't worry. It's never too late to start. You can halt the progressive damage in its tracks and even reverse a lot of it. In this book we will discuss both prevention/protection as well as repairing /correcting.

Chapter 2

Sun Protection

"It is better to prepare and prevent than it is to repair and repent." -
Ezra Taft Benson

Hopefully that last chapter scared you a little bit. We have a problem with the sun. In fact, we have a few problems.

1. Sun damage is a bigger problem than you think.
2. You are probably not protecting yourself well enough.
3. The damage is dramatic and long-lasting.

Disclaimer

I don't want you to completely avoid the sun. I don't want you to stay indoors all the time. Staying inside all day every day can cause bigger problems than sun damage. It's important to go outside. It helps your physical, mental, emotional, and spiritual health to go outside and enjoy what this world has to offer. I want you to go outside, and often. But I want you to be prepared and protected. In this case you CAN have your cake and eat it, too. You can enjoy the outdoors AND still have amazing skin.

An Ounce of Prevention

Benjamin Franklin once said, "An ounce of prevention is worth a pound of cure." Nowhere is it truer than sun exposure and sun damage. In fact, we could do a cost analysis to see if the literal cost of sun protection is actually lower than the literal cost of treating sun damage. Let's do it just for fun.

Cost of yearly aggressive sun protection:
- Liberal use of sunscreen: $20/month = $240/year
- Sun-protective clothing: $30/month = $360/year
  - Total Cost: $50/month = $600/year
  - 10 years = $6,000
  - 20 years = $12,000

Cost of no sun protection:
- Average cost of skin cancer removal: $2000/surgery
- Average number of skin cancers (variable):
- 1-2 cancers/year (sometimes many more)
- Average cost of skin-improving laser procedures: $800/ treatment
- Average number of procedures (variable) 2-4 treatments/year
  - Total cost of reparative treatments: $2,600 - 6,400 per year
  - 10 years = $26,000 - $64,000
  - 20 years = $52,000 - $128,000

Obviously, Ben Franklin was right in this case. Prevention is much more valuable than cure/treatment. Add to that the mental and emotional strains that come from having skin cancers and unhealthy skin. The anxiety and loss of self-confidence can also be very harmful.

Okay, There's a Problem. Now What?

So now we recognize there's a problem, what do we do about it? You're in luck because there's a lot we can do about it. The quote at the beginning of this chapter, "It is better to prepare and prevent than it is to repair and repent" will guide the rest of this book. In this chapter we'll talk about "prepare and prevent." Future chapters will discuss "repair and repent." Prepare and prevent is all about sun protection. The main two categories here are sunscreens and sun-protective clothing. We will delve deeply into those two topics. But first there are a few other sun behavior tips to consider.

Seek the Shade

This may seem obvious, but it is often ignored or neglected. When going outside for a fun activity, simply staying in the shade can be the difference between severe damage and no damage. This is illustrated perfectly if you go to a parade where one side of the street is in shade, and the other side is not. Everyone is watching the same parade for the same amount of time. But it's painfully obvious who's protected and who's getting sun damage. This is easy when it's hot outside. You naturally gravitate toward the shade. But what about when it's not hot outside? You should still seek the shade. Make it a habit. If you pay attention, you'll often find yourself at a bar-b-que, soccer game, swimming pool, walking down a street, or in countless other situations with shade and sun. Seek the shade. It's an easy thing to do and can add up to a big difference over time.

Avoid "Peak Sun"

Peak sunlight happens around mid-day when the sun is the highest. 10 AM to 4 PM is considered the "danger zone" for UV rays. It's also generally the hottest time of the day. This one also seems obvious in the summer when it's hot outside. But you probably don't notice this as much in the spring or fall when the weather is nice. No matter the time of year, the "danger zone" UV rays are many times stronger than other times of the day. There's also less shade available during these times. Sometimes it's out of your control, and you must go out during these times. But sometimes it's not. You can control, for example, when you choose to go to the beach, go on a walk, do your gardening, and many other activities. And if you must go out during the "danger zone," then knowing that you're out at a high-risk time can help you to be more aggressive with your sun protection.

No More Tanning

This one seems obvious, but it can be very challenging, even among people I think already know better. Laying out or going to a tanning bed is just like smoking a cigarette. Period. In fact, this is so important, it bears repeating. Laying out or going to a tanning bed is just like smoking a cigarette. Both cause cancer. Both decrease underlying health and vitality. Both are just plain dangerous. Despite these proven facts, both are still practiced widely. Whenever I go to a beach or swimming pool, I see people laying out. Always. In fact, there are often more people laying out than swimming in the pool or playing at the beach. This is just plain stupid. I've heard all the excuses, too: "I just need a little bit of color," "I need to get my base tan," "I need my vitamin D." These are all lazy arguments and justifications. The truth is that laying out and tanning is an addiction. It causes short-term pleasure and gratification and long-term damage, just like every other addiction. I have seen countless patients now in their 50s, 60s, 70s, and 80s who spent countless hours laying out in their youth. They have terrible skin now--sagging, wrinkled, diseased, and cancerous--all caused by sun damage. They all say the same thing: "In my day we used to lay out with baby oil and mirrors. There was no sunscreen. We didn't know any better." I don't fault them for these behaviors. And I do everything I can to help reverse the damage. But it's often difficult. They would have been much better off to prevent the damage in the first place. They also all say, "I wish I had known better." Well, now we do know better. Now YOU know better. There has never been more knowledge about sun damage and more opportunities for protection. Yet here we are, laying out by the pool.

Sun Protection Strategies

Sun-Protective Clothing

One of the best and most effective options for sun protection is sun-protective clothing. It's a true barrier that prevents the sun from even seeing your skin. It used to be taboo, unfashionable, even laughable to use this approach. Bulky clothing also seems like the last thing you want on a hot summer day. But lately there have been some great advances in sun-protective clothing. There are now many options that are more fashionable, more breathable, more comfortable, and overall, more wearable. Australia is leading the charge in this area. They are dealing with the highest number of skin cancers in the world and have identified this as a major health concern. The Australian government and many private businesses have been working together to increase awareness and provide better protection. This has started to weave itself into the culture of avid nature-lovers and beachgoers. Currently on the beaches of Australia it is commonplace to see people with full-body swimsuits. These are called Stinger Suits and are very effective at blocking UV light. It is also very common to see people outdoors wearing wide-brimmed hats. What Australia is doing is admirable. They're making it fashionable and popular to wear sun-protective clothing.

There are many companies in America that are making these kinds of UV-protective clothing as well. They are made of a tight weave and bear the letters UPF (UV Protective Factor) followed by a number. The number represents how much light is blocked. For example, a UPF of 50 means that 1/50 of light gets through, meaning 2% of light gets through and 98% of light is blocked. This is very effective. It's also very convenient to just put on a hat or long-sleeve shirt and know that it will continually protect your skin: no need to rub it in, and no need to re-apply.

Some companies that specialize in UPF clothing:

- coolibar.com
- Uvskins.com
- Solbari.com
- Solumbra.com

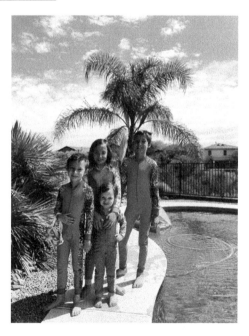

My children wearing their new stinger suits that shipped all the way from Australia.

Sunscreens

Why is it so complicated?

Spoiler alert! Sunscreens work, but you must USE them.

Also, there are some important details to know.

Whenever patients ask me which sunscreen they should use, the conversation goes something like this:

Patient: "Dr. Cope, what sunscreen should I use?"

Me: "Whichever one you like best. "

Patient: "No seriously."

Me: "I'm being serious."

Patient: "Okay then, which one would you recommend?"

Me: "A hat."

The truth is that sunscreens are complicated. Even more complicated is applying them consistently. Most people with a sunburn are people who used sunscreen, but not enough. You're much more likely to use it and use it well when you have a sunscreen that you love. You may say that you don't have a sunscreen you absolutely love. Or, you find the whole sunscreen market confusing and overwhelming. If so, then you're not alone.

Unfortunately, we've taken a simple concept (protect your skin with sunscreen) and made it very confusing with all the packaging, promises, features, risks, and benefits. In this section I will try to educate, simplify, and make recommendations to generally just make your life easier.

Sunscreens can be broken down into two main categories: physical blockers and chemical blockers.

Physical blockers contain zinc and/or titanium as the active ingredient. These are the original sunscreen compounds and they literally block the UV rays from getting to the skin. They work very well at blocking both UVA and UVB. The downside is that they are often thick and pasty. They are hard to rub in and can feel like you are rubbing white paint onto your skin. You sometimes end up looking like a ghost or vampire prepping for Halloween. At least this is traditionally how they have been. Recently there have been some amazing improvements in these sunscreens (more on this later).

Chemical blockers were developed after physical blockers and have become incredibly popular over the last few decades. They are generally cheaper to buy and easier to apply. These contain active ingredients such as oxybenzone, avobenzone, octisalate, octocrylene, homosalate and octinoxate. They work well at absorbing the UV light and preventing it from harming the skin. Until recently, there has been very little concern with chemical sunscreens, and they have been a dominant group. However, in the last few years there have been some legitimate safety concerns that deserve some consideration.

- Absorption - Within the last year of this writing the FDA has performed two studies that show these chemical sunscreen ingredients are being absorbed into the bloodstream from all types of sunscreens (lotions, creams, sprays, and so on). What's more is that they are absorbed in much higher amounts than we ever thought would happen. Do we know what these ingredients are doing inside our bloodstream? No. Not at all. Some have suggested that certain ingredients like oxybenzone may be disrupting hormone functions. However, it could be that there is no damage and no problem. But it sure is concerning for most people to know that sunscreen chemicals are getting absorbed into their blood. This has triggered a lot of interest and concern, and the FDA and other researchers are actively looking into the implications of this.

- Skin reactions - Many people (including me) can develop skin irritation or reactions from the chemicals in chemical sunscreens. When this happens, you basically can't use those ingredients anymore.

- Coral reefs - This is a very hot topic and very politicized right now. Some studies have suggested that chemical sunscreens are harming coral reefs in the form of bleaching. It certainly makes sense that this could happen when millions of people visit a beach wearing chemicals that come off in the water. Over 14,000 tons of sunscreen are estimated to end up in the ocean every year. However, this is very controversial. Some places like Miami Beach, Florida, have rejected these claims, saying there's not enough evidence. Conversely, some places like the state of Hawaii and the republic of Palau have created laws to prevent the use of these sunscreens. The ingredients in question are oxybenzone and octinoxate, both of which are very common in chemical sunscreens.

The MOST Important Thing for Your Skin

Consistency. Just choose a sunscreen and wear it. Every day. Be consistent, just like brushing your teeth. As a doctor, one of the most frustrating things I see is patient non-adherence. I can come up with the correct diagnosis and provide the optimal treatment plan. But the patients will never get better until they actually use the treatment. There is a mountain of research showing that many patients, even a majority, don't ever pick up their prescriptions. And even when they do, they probably don't use it as prescribed. Some fascinating studies with computer chips in the caps of medication bottles showed that patients with severe rashes like eczema and psoriasis didn't use their prescription creams up to 80% of the time! If non-adherence is that bad for patients with diseased and painful skin, imagine how bad it is with sunscreen.

What's the Solution?

Habit and routine. The patients I see with the very best skin (you know, the ones who are 60 and look like they're 40) have been consistently protecting their skin every single day for decades. They don't even think about it anymore. It's just part of the routine, like brushing their teeth. In fact, that's a great time to use sunscreen: right after you brush your teeth. Keep the sunscreen right next to your toothbrush. Every time you brush your teeth just follow it with sunscreen. Other ideas I've seen work well are daily reminders on your smartphone or a daily checklist. Habits are so powerful because you don't have to think about them. They just happen automatically. Good habits strengthen and build you up over time, just as bad habits slowly harm and break you down over time. Your skin will get stronger and healthier over time with good habits. Or it will get weaker, thinner, and older over time--all based on your habits.

SPF: Testing vs. Real Life

Let's assume you defy the odds and you ARE putting on sunscreen every day. One big question remains: Are you wearing enough? If you're like the average person, then you're not. Study after study has shown that most, if not all of us, don't wear enough sunscreen. In fact, you probably put on about half or less of the recommended amount.

When sunscreens are tested in laboratories to get their SPF rating, the amount of sunscreen used is surprisingly high: 2mg/cm². This equates to about 1/2 teaspoon for the entire face, which is a lot more than it seems. When was the last time you put that much sunscreen on your face? Most people are used to putting a pea-sized amount of creams on the face, and that's not even close to what you need. What about the rest of the body? There's a lot of surface area on the back, chest, abdomen, arms, legs, and neck. What about those areas? It would be like bathing in a tub full of sunscreen and then trying to rub it all in.

So, the problems with sunscreen continue. You're probably not putting it on consistently, and not putting on enough. Life is different than the laboratory. In real life, sunscreen is a hassle. An afterthought. Hard to remember. You don't have it when you need it. When you have it, you don't put on enough. And we haven't even talked about the SPF number yet.

(Do you see why my favorite sunscreen is a hat?)

Does SPF number matter?

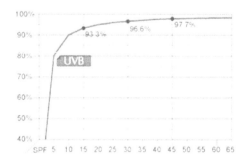

If you look at the percent of UVB blocked by different SPF numbers, you see that it is a logarithmic graph. There is significant increase in coverage between SPF 1 and 10. But after that, increases are small. This has led a lot of people to make the following conclusions over the last few years:

1. There is not much difference between SPF 15 and 30.
2. SPF 30 gives 97% coverage.
3. Improvements beyond SPF 30 are negligible.
4. Therefore, just use sunscreen with SPF 15 or above.

This makes sense when you look at this graph. In fact, the FDA has toyed very seriously with taking away the ability of companies to say anything above SPF 30 or 50. This has been the leading thought for many years, until we remembered one small fact--laboratory conditions are VERY DIFFERENT from real-life conditions. Recently there have been a slew of studies to show that higher SPF sunscreens do, in fact, provide significantly more sun protection than lower SPF sunscreens. This has caused no small stir in the dermatology and sunscreen world. We have been trying to reconcile the above SPF graph with these new findings. And the best we can come up with is this: In the laboratory when we're simply covering probes with large amounts of sunscreen, the UVB blockage does indeed follow this logarithmic graph. But in real life, when we're spreading it over skin using amounts that are much less than the laboratory, the graph looks different. It's unclear how different the graph looks in real life, but my current guess is that it's more like a linear graph than a logarithmic one. So yes, the higher the SPF, the greater the protection.

What About UVA?

One thing that often gets lost in this big discussion about SPF is an enormously important factor: UVA. That's right, UVA isn't even factored into any of this. SPF is specifically a marker of UVB blockage.

And we know that UVA is a major player in damaging your skin. You can block 100% of the UVB in your life and still get thin, wrinkled skin. Thanks, UVA! Luckily, there are sunscreens that effectively block UVA in both the chemical and physical categories. However, currently in America we do not have a formalized way of measuring UVA blockage. We simply have to look for packaging that says, "broad spectrum." Japan has developed a rating system for UVA blockage called the PA+ system (Protection of UVA).

- **PA+** = Some UVA protection
- **PA++** = Moderate UVA protection
- **PA+++** = High UVA protection
- **PA++++** = Extremely High UVA protection

Some companies have started to adopt this PA+ system to test and educate how well their sunscreens block UVA. I applaud them for doing this. Otherwise we're simply left to their packaging and claims. Standardized testing is always preferred, and hopefully we'll get to that point here in America. When in doubt you can look at the ingredients. Zinc (physical blocker) and Avobenzone (chemical blocker) are the two main ingredients that block UVA.

Extra Credit - Oral Supplement

There is an oral supplement called polypodium leucomotomos. It is the extract from a tropical fern plant native to the Americas. There is some evidence that it may in fact help protect your skin from sun damage. This is controversial, and studies have been done to try and see if it is true or not. At this point, some of the studies show that it might work, and some show that it might not work. Either way it is a very safe supplement to take and there is no risk for you to try it. It may help with sun protection and/or repair after sun exposure. But it certainly does not replace the need for more aggressive forms of sun protection.

False Sense of Security

Now you've seen the need for wearing sunscreen, learned about rating systems, committed to physical blockers, and even established a daily routine. You must be all set to never have any sun damage again, right? Wrong! There's a vital piece of information that's still missing, and without it your skin will continue to get fried even when you think it's protected. I'm talking about sunscreen deactivation and the need to re-apply. You've probably heard about this before, and maybe even dismissed it. Unfortunately, it's true. Nearly all sunscreens become deactivated or otherwise ineffective after about 90 minutes. So re-applying is a vital component to complete sun protection. Here's what this looks like in real life.

- Sandra is 45 years old and confident about her sun protection strategy.
- She found a sunscreen that she loves with zinc and titanium.
- She puts it on every morning as part of her routine (it even works as a makeup foundation).
- She is very active throughout the day. Some days she works, and other days she is out and about running errands.
- She knows about sneaky forms of sun exposure like UVA through the windows and "parking lot sun."
- But she feels protected because she puts her sunscreen on every morning at 8 am.

- Sandra comes to see Dr. Cope because there is a new spot on her right temple that's scaly and painful, some dark spots, and some wrinkles that weren't there before.
- She is diagnosed with a new skin cancer, sunspots, and sun-related wrinkling.
- "How can this be?" She exclaims. "I wear sunscreen every day and have for years!"

The problem here is that Sandra didn't realize how important it is to re-apply her sunscreen. It's wonderful that she's been wearing sunscreen every single day. But in some ways, this has become problematic for her. It has created a false sense of security. By putting on sunscreen at 8 am, she felt comfortable outside in the sun at 12 pm when the sun is at its most intense. She relied on that 8 am application, when actually, it was long gone. It's like the emperor's new clothes. He thought he was well-dressed for the parade. But actually, he was naked.

The importance of re-applying can't be overstated. It can also be very challenging to accomplish. How do you reapply sunscreen at work or in your car, when the tube is at home in your drawer? The best answer I have found is to have multiple tubes of your favorite sunscreen. If it's nearby, you'll use it. If you hide it or hoard it, you won't. Keep one at home, one in your car, one in your purse, and one at work. Just find a combination that works well for you and your life. Keep something always nearby that you can use when you need it. A quick application before you leave work or leave the restaurant will make a huge difference in your skin over time.

My Favorite Products

"What product should I use?" Or "Dr. Cope, what's your favorite sunscreen?" These are the questions that invariably arise after a discussion of sunscreens. I'll give my current favorite products, recognizing that this is an industry with many players and a lot of innovation. Therefore, my favorites evolve over time based on what I think are the best options. I also recommend a hat, long sleeves, and the sun-avoidance behaviors mentioned above to every patient.

Here are my current favorites, in no particular order.

Physical Blocking Sunscreens

Note that this is my preferred category of sunscreens. They are overall safer and more effective. They are generally more expensive as well.

- Colorescience Sunforgettable Total Protection Face Shield (SPF 50, PA+++) - This is a very nice, easy to apply, physical blocking sunscreen. Colorescience is an impressive company. They make nothing but physical blocking sunscreens that are practical, easy to use, and work extremely well. They have impressive Enviroscreen technology that also traps and minimizes free radicals.
- Colorescience Sunforgettable Brush-on Shield (SPF 50, PA++++) - This is the most convenient product I've ever seen. It's a powder that you brush on to your skin. It is so easy to apply. My kids love it and call it "the magic brush." You can put it on top of make-up or anything else you have on your skin. It is also the easiest to re-apply. It's tinted, but goes on clear.
- Sunbetter Sheer Sunscreen Stick by SkinBetter (SPF 56) - I love sunscreen sticks because they are also easy to apply. You still have

to rub them in, but they just seem less messy and more convenient. This is a high-quality product that I also put on my kids when we go hiking. Just don't leave it in the car or it can liquify. Zinc and Titanium.

- Essential Defense Mineral Shield by Skin Medica (SPF 35, PA++++) - This is a simple, easy to use, easy to rub in sunscreen. It doesn't run and it works well. It is clear (non-tinted)
- Elta MD UV Physical (SPF 41) - This one is tinted. It rubs on easily. It comes in a large tube and is well-priced.

Chemical Sunscreens

These are currently under fire for reasons mentioned earlier. But they do have some great redeeming features. They're cheaper and easier to use. Plus, they work. We don't know if they're really doing any damage in the blood or in the coral reefs; this is the controversy. But there is no controversy over the fact that direct sunlight will destroy your skin. So, if it comes down to chemical sunscreen or nothing, I'd choose chemical sunscreen every time.

- Neutrogena Ultra Sheer Dry Touch (SPF 100) - An SPF 100 for less than $10. That's pretty interesting if you ask me.
- Elta 46 Clear Broad Spectrum (SPF 46) - This is a very nice sunscreen that is so incredibly easy to put on. Even my father (who hates sunscreen) doesn't mind putting this one on. It's very popular among dermatology offices and patients.
- La Roche-Posay Anthelios Melt-in Sunscreen Milk (SPF 60) - This one has come out on top of Consumer Reports' sunscreen testing (laboratory- based testing) for many years running. It is consistently a high-quality product.

- Trader Joe's Spray (SPF 50) – Again, a high-quality spray that consistently tests among the best with Consumer Reports testing. Interestingly, the chemical sunscreens always seem to do better than physical blockers in the Consumer Reports testing. They keep their testing methods very "hush hush" though because it's a proprietary process.
- Walgreens Hydrating Lotion (SPF 50). If you're looking for the best "bang for your buck," this is it. $3 for a sunscreen that is proven to be very effective is a bargain (again by Consumer Reports testing). It also does not contain any oxybenzone.

Chapter 3

Topical Skincare Products

What is All This Stuff?

The topical over the counter (OTC) skincare market in the US is massive and complicated. If you were confused by sunscreens, then you're likely flabbergasted by skincare. There are so many options: creams, ointments, serums, ceramides, exfoliators, toners, acids, peels, and so on. And the packaging promises everything from baby-perfect skin all the way to the planet Jupiter. The prices are also confusing. Should you get the most expensive creams? Does a higher price mean they're better? What are these things made of, liquified gold nuggets? Are you confused or skeptical? Don't worry, so is everyone else. The purpose of this chapter is to try and clarify this mess of topical skincare products. I want you to be able to understand the most important categories and be confident that you have exactly the products you need--no more and no less. There's a strategy for everyone. Are you on a budget? Are you a minimalist? Do you want the best of the best? Do you want the best skin humanly possible? Don't worry, there's a topical strategy for all these options.

Do I Really Need to Put on Topicals?

Do you really need topical products for your skin? Only if you want great skin. And only if you want skin that stays great for years and years. I've seen many older patients with terrible skin (especially during my stint working at the VA). But I've also seen some older patients with incredible skin (even if they have a history of sun exposure). Naomi is a patient of mine who regularly comes in for skin checks and small maintenance procedures. She has amazing skin and looks much younger than she really is. The first time I met Naomi I didn't look at her age in her chart. I just started chatting with her and getting to know her. I asked where she worked, and she told me she'd been working as an office manager at a nearby medical practice for 30 years.

"Wait a minute," I said. "How have you been working there for 30 years when you look like you're in your 30s?"

Well, as it turned out, Naomi was 58 and had indeed been working in the same job for 30 years. I was blown away. Since then, I've seen many more patients just like Naomi, who look decades younger than their true age. What do they all have in common? Two things:

1) A consistent routine of using high quality topical products.

2) Regular checkups 2-3x/year for skin checks and small maintenance procedures (more on these later).

So yes, if you want to have great skin, then you need to have a great topical product program. We'll get into each of the products and make this as simple and manageable as possible. But first and foremost, we need to discuss (again) an incredibly important point — habit and routine. Yes, our old friend habit from the last chapter is here to pester us again. The unfortunate truth about these topicals is this: The best products in the world will do NOTHING unless you actually USE THEM. I'm sorry if this seems trivial, repetitive, or elementary. But the sad truth is that most people (and certainly most of the people I see) don't reliably use their topical products. There's only so much I can do for these people. It's like trying to remove a splinter in the dark, or clear a swamp full of mosquitos with a single can of bug spray. It's a losing battle. I can't emphasize enough the importance of using your topicals every day. Consistently. Religiously. Otherwise, we're wasting our time.

Prevention AND Correction

The good news is that once you nail down your daily routine and get the right products, you can simultaneously provide **prevention and correction** to your skin. That's right: prevention AND correction at the same time! The skin is an incredible living organ. With a little work we can help it to help itself. It can become stronger, thicker, and more protective. This also gives you a more youthful appearance.

Realistic Expectations

When the aging process is reversed, your skin can start to correct itself from the inside out. You can get significant improvement from previous sun damage (wrinkles, sunspots, pre-cancerous lesions, and so on). These benefits can be dramatic, but they are also slow and steady. You won't see dramatic results in just a couple of days. There will also be side effects to put up with (nothing worth having comes without some effort). It's hard on your skin to undergo some of these changes. It's very common to have some dryness, peeling, and redness for the first few weeks. This is very normal and actually means that the topicals are working. It's important for you to be aware of this process. I've had patients stop their products because they think they're having an allergic reaction or getting a burn. I have to remind them that all is well and this is what's supposed to happen.

The Skin is Like a Muscle

Muscle and skin have a lot in common. They can both get better and stronger, but it's a difficult process and causes some discomfort along the way. When you lift weights, your muscles develop micro tears. This is what causes soreness for the next few days. As the muscles heal, they become stronger to be able to better withstand this kind of strain. This is why you can lift heavier and heavier amounts of weight, and why the original weight no longer causes soreness afterward. Skin, like muscle, responds to external forces. The equivalent of lifting weights for your skin is daily application of certain products. These provide minor stress and strain to the skin. The result is that the skin gets stronger. It does this by speeding up the skin cycle of developing new cells and shedding old/dead cells. This is why you get red and scaly when you first start. Eventually the skin gets used to this continual strain and is better and stronger because of it.

The Problem With Moisturizer

Let's continue this muscle analogy. If certain topicals strengthen the skin and help it to get in shape, then too much moisturizer does the opposite. It's like making the skin fat and lazy, like preventing your muscles from exercising, which leads to wasting and atrophy. This is because the skin moisturizes itself from the inside out. If your skin is healthy and disease-free, then it should be producing all the moisturizer that it needs from inside. When you put a lot of moisturizer over the top from the outside in, the skin gets the message that it doesn't need to produce anything from the inside out. It shuts off the feedback loop. So, your skin gets lazy. Lazy skin has less thickness, provides less protection, and has less vitality. What you need to do is slap your skin a little bit. Help it wake up. Help it to start to work for you again. We do this by giving it signals to strengthen itself. Is there a role for moisturizer? Yes, but it's likely different from what you've been taught in the past.

The Perfect Skin Regimen

It's impossible to perfectly tailor a skin regimen to you without seeing your skin in-person. But there are some principles that apply to most people. Important components include the following:

- Washing system (cleanser, scrub, and toner)
- Retinoid
- Antioxidants
- Pigment controllers
- Exfoliators

We'll cover each of these categories in depth. And at the end of the chapter, I'll show you two possible daily regimens (including morning and night applications).

Cleanser, Scrub, and Toner

A strong system of facial washing, scrubbing, and toning is critical. It's the warm-up and stretching for all your skin workouts. You can't have beautiful, young, and smooth skin without it. This is step number one in the morning and at night. It makes every subsequent step work better. The three steps together work synergistically as well.

1. Cleanser - Removes dirt, pollution, oils, and impurities from your skin. These are damaging your skin and preventing proper exfoliation of the dead skin cells and absorption of the important products.

2. Scrub or polish – This is a little more aggressive (don't get too frisky here) and helps to exfoliate the skin. Removing the top layer of dead skin cells is very important. It stimulates the feedback loop and sends signals to the deeper layers to continue producing healthy and strong skin. Removing layers of dead cells also helps your next layers of topical products to absorb much better.

3. Toner - These are usually pads, sometimes with a fruity smell. They often contain a gentle acid that changes the pH of your skin. The ideal pH of your skin is slightly acidic (vs. slightly basic). This helps your skin to again have optimal conditions for health and strength. Acidic skin also helps with acne and other skin diseases. And it provides a better environment for absorption of other products.

Favorite Skin Washes

- ZO "Getting Skin Ready" - washing system
- Skin Better oxygen infusion wash
- Revision Wash

Retinoids (My Favorite Category)

I can't say enough about this category. After sunscreen I see it as THE most important category of topical skin care. And the primary reason I suggest a strong washing system is to help the retinoid to get better absorption. Retinoids are a family of chemicals that go by various names: retinol, Retin-A (brand name), tretinoin, retinoic acid. They are all derivatives of vitamin A. If you have ever used the oral acne medication Accutane (isotretinoin), these compounds are basically the cream version of Accutane. Retinoids work as transcription factors for your skin. That means they go deep into the nucleus of each cell and stimulate certain receptors to start transcribing certain sections of DNA. The long-term effect is that you get faster growth and turnover of the skin, which leads to healthier and younger skin. This is the true exercising of your skin, or the "heavy lifting." If you use a retinoid every day for weeks/months/years, then you will eventually have the "body builder" level of skin. Your skin will look great no matter how old you are. You will consistently look younger than people your same chronological age. It will also prevent skin cancer, stimulate collagen, treat and prevent acne, prevent wrinkles, and even decrease wrinkles you already have. If anything could be considered a "miracle cream," then it's the retinoids.

Common Side Effects

I know what you're thinking. These retinoids sound too good to be true. And you're right. There are some side effects that you need to know about. Not serious side effects, just annoying. It's mostly redness, dryness, and peeling. The good news is that these are temporary. After the first few weeks your skin starts to get used to this "new normal," and the side effects tend to go away. To some people these side effects are not so bad, and they can get through it knowing that great benefits are in store. But for some people, these side effects are just too much, and they stop using the cream. Others get worried and think they're having an allergic reaction. You can see that mental prepping for this redness and peeling is a very important step.

Another important discussion is how to deal with the sun. While on a retinoid your skin will become more sensitive to the sun. This isn't necessarily a bad thing as it may help you to commit to daily sun protection more fully. Also, direct sunlight will deactivate the cream, so we tell people to use it at night. As you can see, it takes a lot of time to fully have this discussion with your dermatologist, and sometimes it gets skipped or abbreviated. You need to know beforehand what's going to happen and how to deal with it.

Coping Strategies

If you're struggling with these common side effects, here are a few coping strategies to help you get through it.

- **Start Gently** - There are hundreds (if not thousands) of products in this retinoid category. Some are very gentle, and some are very strong, with everything in between. You may want to start with a gentler product and slowly graduate to stronger products. Note that it is very important to eventually get to the stronger products to get the maximum benefit. Some people forget this and stay with the weak/gentle version for years without getting the full benefit of the retinoid. To be fair, something is better than nothing, but the biggest benefit comes from the strongest products.

- **Start Every Other Day** – This allows your skin to slowly acclimate to the new product. You can do this for a few weeks then slowly increase to every day. Note that it is very important to eventually get up to every day. Again, I have seen people stay at every other day for years. They have minimal side effects, but they are not getting the full benefit.

- **Grin and Bear It (My favorite)** - This can be tough, but it seems to be the best option for most people. It's for people who understand and want the full benefit of the cream. They are paying good money for it and they want the full result. They start with a strong cream and use it every day. They have redness, scaling, sometimes tingling, but they know it's temporary. Then, after a few weeks this has all resolved and they quickly start to notice dramatic improvement in their skin tone and texture and quality. It also helps them to fully commit, and the extra challenges further drive home that commitment.

Favorite Products
- ZO Radical Night Repair
- ZO Wrinkle & Texture Repair
- SkinBetter AlphaRet
- Skin Medica Retinol
- Altreno lotion (tretinoin .05%) - Rx only
- Generic tretinoin (.05% or .1%) - Rx only

What About Pigment Problems?

Dyspigmentation is a very common problem. It can be especially noticeable for people with darker skin types. When you're young your melanocytes create a nice uniform pigment throughout all the skin cells. The result is a nice uniform tan. As we age, though, the uniformity is lost. The pigment gets dispersed haphazardly and becomes blotchy. You may notice a sunspot or two or develop melasma.* Basically, if you tan your skin when you're young, then you'll probably get some blotchy dyspigmentation when you're older (starting in your 30s). Once again, it's better to prepare and prevent than to repair and repent.

*Note - If you ever have questions or concerns about dark spots on your skin, you're never wrong to have them looked at by a dermatologist. It's always important to rule out melanoma in these cases.

Pigment Controllers

If you've started to notice some dyspigmentation in your skin, then it's probably time to add some pigment controllers to your topical regimen. These are also known as "bleaching creams" and are an essential component of treatment for pigment disorders. Most of these products use a medication called hydroquinone as the active ingredient. This is a prescription medication and warrants an important discussion with a dermatologist as well. There are also other pigment- improving products that use other active ingredients, but none work as well as hydroquinones. The way these work is by basically blocking the pigment production pathway from tyrosine to melanin. This is reversible and only works if you're using the medication. This halting of pigment production is very helpful in combination with a strong retinoid that is actively exfoliating the skin and gets rid of current pigment. This same idea applies to chemical peels and laser treatments to remove the top layers.

Side Effects

Hydroquinones can work amazingly well, but they also have some side effects to be aware of. These are generally skin irritation, redness, peeling, and itching. Many of these are similar to the retinoid side effects and often tend to get better in the same timeframe. There are also two different kinds of paradoxical hyperpigmentation that can happen with too much hydroquinone use. The first is feedback loop overproduction. This happens when the melanocytes start to wake up and try to produce extra pigment. This generally happens when someone is using their hydroquinone sporadically over a long period of time (years). It can be avoided if used correctly. The other is a very rare and very challenging condition called exogenous ochronosis. This is where a different kind of pigment, usually blue/grey in color, happens on the face. It is a buildup of a chemical called homogentisic acid. This is very rare and typically happens in people who use very high concentrations of hydroquinones for a very long time. It also generally happens in darker skin types. These side effects are the reason why this medication requires a prescription and should be managed by a dermatologist.

The Best Strategy

I've found the best strategy for using hydroquinones is the following:

- Use hydroquinone daily for 2-3 months (basically until the tube runs out of cream). Note that I don't often go very high on the strength, to be on the safe side.
- After 2-3 months, switch to another method of pigment control.
- Alternate these two methods every 3 months or so.

Pre-Laser Skin Prep

It's also important to know about skin prep for any traumatic facial procedure. All skin types, but especially darker skin types, can develop hyperpigmentation after trauma to the skin. It's called post-inflammatory hyperpigmentation (PIH). This happens after rashes, acne, and injury. It can also happen after a laser procedure, Microneedling, benign growth removal, skin surgery, and so on. For this reason, it is very important to prep the skin with a retinoid and hydroquinone prior to any skin procedures. This helps to prevent PIH and optimize the outcome of these treatments. I put all my procedure patients on a skin prep regimen for 2-4 weeks prior to the procedure.

Favorite Pigment Products
1. ZO Pigment Control
2. ZO Pigment Control + Blending
3. Rx Hydroquinone (compounded)

What are Antioxidants?

You've probably heard the word *antioxidants*, and unless you're a scientist or physician you were initially confused as to what these are and what they do. You could spend a lot of time studying free radicals and antioxidants (and some very smart people do exactly that). In a nutshell, free radicals are high energy molecules that can cause damage to surrounding cells. Often that damage results in the death of the surrounding cells. In the skin this contributes to the chronic thinning of the skin you see with age. Free radicals are produced by UV light, pollution, and even normal visible light (blue light is the biggest problem here and is very abundant in the light from screens). These free radicals often do their damage in the dermis, where they kill the fibroblasts and destroy collagen and elastin. They can continue to wreak havoc for up to three hours after sun exposure. Free radicals need to be addressed, and the way to address them is with antioxidants.

Antioxidants help to calm down free radicals from their highly energized state through exchanging electrons. Applying antioxidants to your skin helps to reduce the damage caused by free radicals that are generated throughout the day. Your body produces its own antioxidants, but these can become overwhelmed and sometimes need a little extra help. Antioxidants can also help to increase the actual UV protection of the skin and can improve DNA repair processes. That's a lot of great benefits to your skin. Overall, antioxidants are a great addition to a good daily skin care regimen.

Some popular antioxidant ingredients are described below.

- Vitamin C - This is the most well known and most popular antioxidant. It works well and is included in many products. It has a lot of great benefits, too (free radical repair, UV protection, DNA repair). The downside is that it's hard to stabilize the molecule into a topical product (you often see it in a serum or anhydrous dry cream), and there are some side effects that can occur (skin irritation and acne).

- Niacinamide - This antioxidant is a variant of vitamin B3, or niacin. While niacin can cause redness and flushing (in pill form), niacinamide can do the opposite and actually reduce redness. In pill form as a supplement it can also help prevent skin cancers, and potentially it can help with this in topical form as well.

Favorite Products

- Skinceuticals CE Ferrulic
- Skinceuticals Fluoritin CF (for acne prone skin)
- ZO Daily Power & Defense
- SkinBetter Alto Defense - 19 antioxidants, niacinamide to reduce redness, no breakouts (even though it has Vitamin C)
- Skin MedicaTotal Defense & Repair
- Colorescience Enviroscreen Products
- Skin Medica TNS Advanced+

Exfoliators

These are products that speed up and increase the amount of exfoliation. The retinoids are the primary exfoliators as we discussed previously. But these guys help your skin to increase and speed up this process. They basically amplify the benefits of the retinoids, leading to healthier skin, thicker collagen, and younger appearance. The main ingredients here are different weak acids (glycolic, lactic, and others).

Favorite Products

- Exfoliation Accelerator
- Alpharet Intensive (Retinol that adds glycolic)

A Role for Moisturizers

Moisturizers are so common, they could have an entire state or two named after them. They are common, but as discussed above, they are probably doing more harm than good by making your skin lazy and unproductive. We need to kick the skin into gear and help it to produce its own moisturizer. But we need to know when to help the skin from the outside-in while it strengthens from the inside-out. There are many nuances to this discussion, but here's a good rule of thumb for you. Use moisturizer in these three situations: When the skin is injured, scabbed, or the barrier is impaired (red and peeling). This barrier problem is the most common and can happen temporarily when you're first starting your aggressive skin regimen. It also happens with many different types of rashes. (So this advice might be helpful for your next rash.)

Which Moisturizer Should You Use?

You want to find a moisturizer that helps the most and has the lowest chance of causing problems. Here are two simple rules to follow.

- Avoid anything with fragrance. If it smells nice, then don't put it on your skin. Fragrances are some of the most common culprits for contact allergic dermatitis. Even if you don't have a skin allergy to these things, you can develop one later. It's just smarter to steer clear of fragrant lotions and creams.

- The thicker the better. Thin lotions that come out of a pump are almost always too thin. They often contain alcohols or glycerin, things that can irritate and even dry out your skin. The thickest and best thing you can put on your skin is 100% pure petroleum jelly. That's right. The thick gooey stuff. It will make you feel greasy and shiny, but it's by far the best. It basically seals the skin barrier and helps trap the skin's own moisture inside, rather than letting it get out of the impaired barrier. Ointments are thicker than creams. Creams are thicker than lotions. If you want to use a cream, it should come in a jar with a big lid that needs to come off to use it, not a pump.

Favorite Products

- Vaseline - It's the oldest, most well-known brand of 100% petroleum jelly. It just works. Period. You can use any generic version that may be a little cheaper, too. You may be concerned that Vaseline will clog pores and cause acne. This is more dogma than actual science. Studies have not found this to be the case.

- Aquaphor - This is a little less greasy than Vaseline, so some people prefer this. If you buy in to the "Vaseline clogs pores" idea, then this one is less likely to do that since it's a lower percentage of petroleum jelly. It's also a little more expensive.

- Cerave - This is a nice thick cream. If you just can't stand the above ointments, then try this cream. It has ceramides that help to absorb into the skin and help it to repair.
- Cetaphil - Another good cream option; it's very basic and devoid of a lot of filler-chemicals (a really good thing).

Simple Plan vs 100%

Chances are that as you're reading about these topical products, you're falling into one of two camps.

- Camp 1: "Wow, this all sounds amazing. I want to get all these benefits. I want great skin, and I'm willing to work for it. I want to do it all!"
- Camp 2: "Wow, this all sounds overwhelming. I can't do all of this. I'd rather do nothing than try to keep up with all this stuff. I can maybe handle putting one or two things on my face each day."

No matter what camp you fall into, you can create a plan and a system that works for you. It's so much better to do something rather than nothing. You need to find a system that works for you and stick with it.

If you find yourself in Camp 1 and gung-ho, then go for it! Remember that sticking with it over time is the most important thing, so don't burn out.

If, on the other hand, you find yourself in Camp 2, then listen up. Don't get discouraged or overwhelmed. Many (in fact most) people are in this camp. And unfortunately, most of them just end up doing nothing and their skin suffers. You're probably looking for the simplest program that provides the most benefit, or the most "bang for your buck." Below is the simple program that does exactly that. It's the 80/20 of daily skin care (20% of products yields 80% of the results).

Simple Plan

- AM - Wash and Sunscreen
- PM - Wash and Retinol (pea size for entire face)

100% Plan

- AM
  - Wash and Scrub (likely in the shower)
  - Pigment corrector
  - Exfoliation accelerator
  - Antioxidant
  - Aggressive Sun Protection (re-apply throughout the day)
- PM
  - Wash and Toner
  - Enzymatic peel
  - Pigment corrector (can be mixed with retinol)
  - Strong Retinol (use 2-3x more than pea-size)

Stick With It

No matter what you do, there will be some side effects. It's minimal with the simple plan, but it's still there. With the 100% plan it can be dramatic (my wife said her skin was "snowing"). Stick with it! You're working out your skin. Trust the process. Trust your "personal trainer." This will work, and you'll be grateful for your great skin.

A Dermatologist's Story

I know a very prominent dermatologist who tells a story about when he was dating his wife. He started her on a very aggressive topical skin program for six weeks. He explained that it would be tough for those six weeks, but the benefits would be amazing. But he didn't stop there. He knew she would be very red and peeling, so he tried to keep her motivated. He sent her roses every single day for those six weeks as a reminder that she was doing great and it would all be worth it. They both tell this story to this day with big smiles on their faces (and great skin).

Chapter 4

Skin Lasers

At a Glance

1. Lasers are amazing technology with a diverse range of functions in the skin.

2. The most common lasers are those that help remove or soften wrinkles.

3. Just about everyone over the age of 30 probably needs a laser treatment of some sort.

4. Some are much stronger and require significant down time.

5. Some are gentle with minimal downtime but need more treatment sessions

6. Some are in-between (Goldilocks) with less downtime but still noticeable results.

7. Once you have great skin and are on a maintenance program you should still do a laser 1-2x per year.

8. Get lasers done at a reputable medical practice, one that knows the skin well and will be safe with their lasers.

What are Lasers?

Lasers are an incredible new technology. They can do amazing things for the skin on the face. From wrinkles to brown spots, to red skin and red vessels, there's virtually something for everyone. The problem with lasers is that they can be confusing. In recent years there has been an explosion of new lasers and many new companies popping up to create them. It's gotten to the point where you really need someone who understands lasers to take you by the hand and explain everything. Lasers can also be dangerous. They can cause burns and skin pigment problems. They can even cause blindness (if misfired into the eyes). Lasers are very important for an optimal treatment and maintenance regimen for your skin, so it's worth it to find a place that safely delivers effective treatments. If you want healthy skin, then you need to include lasers in your life. But you definitely want someone operating the laser who knows how to use it and how to keep you safe.

How do Lasers Work?

Each laser has a substance inside known as the "medium." Light energy passes through the medium and produces a very specific wavelength of light. This specific wavelength targets a very specific component of tissue called a chromophore. The three main chromophores in the skin are hemoglobin (for red lasers), melanin (for pigment lasers), and water (for resurfacing lasers). Some lasers can also target the different colors of tattoos. When the laser hits the target chromophore, it causes it to vibrate and/or heat up to a point where it kills the cell. But only the cells containing the target chromophore are killed. This is called selective photothermolysis. In the case of water as the chromophore, the laser hits the water inside the top layer of cells and kills those cells, allowing for a "laser resurfacing" to occur. There are many other details and nuances about the physics of lasers, but this basic overview is all you really need to understand at this point.

Lasers also differ in the amounts of energies that are used. This is important because certain skin types (generally darker and more pigmented) are more sensitive to lasers and can have bad reactions if too much energy is used.

The Laser Gamut: Super Strong to Very Gentle

The most common reason you might want to use a laser is to reduce or minimize the wrinkles on your face. There is a wide range of lasers you can choose from to do this job. These range from an aggressive "one and done" experience, to very gentle "lunchtime lasers," and everything in between.

The strongest lasers correspond to the best results, highest cost, and most downtime. This is also called fully ablative resurfacing. The biggest players here are CO2 lasers and erbium lasers.

The gentlest lasers have very little to no downtime, are cheaper, and require multiple sessions to get the desired result. Even after multiple treatments they will never give you a result as good as an aggressive CO2 or erbium laser. But that might be perfect for you.

And then you get the in-between or "Goldilocks" lasers that can give you the best of both worlds. They're not too strong, and not too gentle. They can produce a very good result with less downtime. Everything is in between the other categories: results, downtime, and cost. For many people this is the perfect category. They can tolerate the discomfort and downtime and are still happy with the end results. This category is especially popular for people who can't get much time off from work.

Stronger Lasers

The strongest lasers are also the most challenging recoveries, requiring the most downtime and the most aftercare. But nothing produces a better result than these ultra-strong lasers. If you have significant sun damage, this is the answer for you. It can really take away 5 to 10 years of aging and sun damage from your skin. But you need to know how challenging this process can be. For the first few days don't look in the mirror. You will look like a burn victim. You will not like what you see. And you must stay completely out of the sun. Don't even get close to it. This can cause problems like hyperpigmentation. Take the after-care steps seriously. Keep the ointment on your face, wash gently and regularly, and protect your skin from the sun. You'll likely never need to do this again, and you probably won't want to. Once it's all healed your skin will look better and feel better than ever. It will even remove some superficial growths, including pre-cancerous ones. Examples of strong resurfacing lasers include Lumenis Ultrapulse (CO2) and Fotona SP Dynamis (Erbium)

Gentle Lasers

On the other end of the spectrum are the gentle lasers. These only target the most superficial layers of skin. They create a nice glow for a few days and weeks. These effects are not permanent though, as the skin continues to turnover and go through its regular processes. The downtime is easy, with only a light pink for a day or two, and maybe some light peeling. You will need a series of these treatments to get any lasting and noticeable effects. Examples of these lasers are Clear and Brilliant and IPL (more for discoloration but helps with texture too). I have seen some people with wonderful skin who attribute their success to these lasers. They come in virtually every month for a procedure and don't do anything else. It's a true "lunchtime laser" scenario that only takes an hour or so, then you can get back to work or life. These can work well, but you must commit to getting them done regularly. Some celebrities say they do exclusively these types of lasers for their skin, and they have great skin.

"Goldilocks" Lasers

In between the ultra-strong and gentler lasers live the "Goldilocks" lasers. These are the ones that aren't too strong and aren't too weak. There's less downtime, but still good results. The price is also generally squarely in the middle. You may be thinking, "I want to do a laser treatment, but I don't want my face to look like it's falling off for the first week, and I don't have a full week to stop living my life and stay cooped up like a hermit." Perhaps you're thinking, "I want to do a laser treatment, but I don't want to keep coming back every month for 6-10 months to finally start seeing a result. I'm paying good money for this, so I want to see some results ASAP." If these statements resonate with you, then a "Goldilocks" laser is probably the laser for you. These lasers are strong and effective, but generally fractionated. This means they only treat a percentage of the skin rather than the entire surface area. It's somewhat like aerating your lawn and taking out little plugs. This strategy helps with the health of your lawn and it helps with the health of your skin. The downtime is generally not severe. You'll have a deep red sunburn-look and a few days of peeling after that. You may need to repeat the treatment 2-3 times to get the optimal result. Another benefit is that these lasers are generally safer for darker skin types. Examples of good "Goldilocks" lasers are Fotona Micropeel, Fraxel Dual, and Halo by Sciton.

Reds and Browns

There are also lasers that target specific colors in the skin. The biggest targets here are the reds and browns. Reds are generally caused by overgrowth of superficial blood vessels. And browns are generally caused by overproduction of pigment. These discolorations can lead to an overall skin appearance that is aged and distracting, even if the skin itself is healthy. By targeting these specific colors, laser treatments can restore a more uniform coloring to the skin. The big players here are vascular lasers (excel V by Cutera, Vbeam by Candela), IPL (intense pulsed light), PicoSure by Cynosure and other pigment-specific lasers. These lasers do not ablate the tissue on the outside. They target the specific chromophore within and help to break up the color or structure which then gets eliminated over time. These are great lasers that are very helpful to the overlying picture of the skin. Depending on what you're trying to accomplish, you will probably need multiple treatments with these lasers.

Other Options

There are many players in the laser and skin treatment game. Some are similar, substitutes, or good add-on procedures. But most of them would not be considered true lasers.

- Microneedling - This is a category that is taking off in popularity. It is like a gentle laser in that there's low downtime. It's also generally cheaper than most lasers for anti-aging, or acne scarring. It also requires a series of 3-6 treatments to get good results.

- PRP - This is an exciting technology that often works in combination with laser. PRP stands for Platelet-Rich-Plasma. You get your own blood drawn and spun down. Then we take just the liquid portion (plasma) that also contains the platelets. These get activated and release many different growth factors into the tissue. This can be helpful for healing tissue (joint injections), hair growth (hair loss injections), or anti-aging (skin drizzling after laser procedure).

- Radio Frequency (RF) Microneedling - There are many different RF devices out there. They are as vast and varied as our Milky Way galaxy. They generally treat a little deeper and can help with skin tightening. I have seen some amazing results and some terrible results (and complications) with RF devices. I know that many people use them and swear by them. I personally am not terribly impressed by the consistency of results and the cost for patients. I think there are things that work better, and for the time-being, those are the things I'm recommending for my patients.

What About Chemical Peels?

This is a great place to talk about peels, since they can accomplish a lot of the same things that lasers can. In fact, some of the best results I've ever seen have been from a chemical peel. When choosing between a laser and a chemical peel, it basically comes down to a trade-off. Chemical peels are cheaper, and they still can work very well. The downside is that they can be more painful, and it can be hard to control the depth, so you may have a higher risk of complications. On the other side, lasers tend to be more expensive but have more control over their depth (very precise). There's also the question of availability. Specific lasers may be hard to come by in your area, while chemical peels tend to be more common in medical practices. There's no right or wrong when it comes to chemical peels vs. laser, just different pros and cons to consider. There are many dermatologists who will combine the two together in amazing and creative ways to deliver fantastic results.

Possible Adverse Effects

All lasers basically have the same potential complications and adverse effects. However, it's important to know that proper medical workup, preparation, and technique can dramatically reduce the risk of these (if not prevent them entirely). These potential complications are burns, eye injury, infection, pigment problems, and persistent redness

- Burns - This can happen when a laser's energy is too strong for a specific skin type, or when the laser operator lingers too long on a specific area. This can generally be prevented with proper training (correct energies and correct technique).

- Eye Injury - Every laser can cause severe eye injury if fired directly into the eyes. For this reason, you must wear eye shields during every laser procedure. And everyone else in the room needs to wear appropriate eye protection provided by the clinic.

- Infection - Lasers that ablate the skin create a risk for bacteria to get introduced and cause infection. This can slow down healing and increase the risk of scarring. This can be prevented with a high-quality and detailed post-care program. Infection can also be identified early and effectively treated to prevent problems.

- Pigment problems - Lasers can cause HYPERpigmentation (extra pigment production) or rarely HYPOpigmentation (less pigment production) of the skin. The extra pigment production is the most common. In fact, this happens any time the skin gets inflamed, especially in darker skin types. It's called post-inflammatory hyperpigmentation (PIH). We often see it in patients with acne that leaves behind dark spots. You may think this is scarring, but it's not--just too much pigment which eventually fades. The good news about PIH and laser is that it can be prevented. Certain lasers we avoid completely with darker skin types. But others can work just fine. This is why I pre-treat every laser patient with hydroquinone and retinoids.

- Persistent redness - Rarely after a laser will you have an area of treated skin that stays red for a long time. This generally happens with stronger lasers and in people who tend to hold on to red for a variety of reasons. This can be prevented with a good skin prep protocol. And it can be treated (ironically enough) with another laser--the red or vascular lasers.

Worth the Trouble

I know it can be concerning to read about all the possible side effects. But just know that these are very rare, especially in a high-quality medical practice. When lasers are used safely and correctly, they can do incredible things for your skin. And if you have significant sun damage, then laser may be your best (and only) option for significant improvement.

Chapter 5

Dynamic Lines and Botox

Dynamic Lines

Dynamic lines are the lines between your eyebrows, the lines on your forehead, and the lines by your eyes when you squint. They're called dynamic lines because they happen when you move your underlying facial muscles. They are rare to see in young skin (babies and children), but as you get older you start to notice them more and more. The reason they become more pronounced over time is because of sun damage. The sun causes skin thinning, which is less able to resist the underline movements. The facial muscles can also get stronger over time as you use them more. As a result, these lines get deeper, longer, and more pronounced as you age. Eventually they look more like furrows or creases, and they can be seen even at rest.

What Can we Do About It?

The main solution for these dynamic lines is Botox. Actually, the correct term is neuromodulator (or neurotoxin) and one of the more famous of the neuromodulator medications is brand-named Botox. In this case, the brand Botox has become synonymous with neuromodulator, so we often use these interchangeably. There are 3-4 other brands of neuromodulators in the US currently, with more coming in the future. Other options are Dysport, Xeomin, and Jeaveau, and they all do pretty much the same thing (with some very subtle differences.)

Neuromodulators

Botox and its competitors have become very popular over the last few years and have proven to be very safe and effective. Virtually everyone has at least heard about Botox, but very few seem to understand what it is and what it does. Initially there was a bit of a negative stigma about Botox among those who didn't know much about it. But this negative stigma seems to be improving over the last few years.

Botox is a molecule called onabotulinumtoxinA (a mouthful, I know). It is derived from the bacterium clostridium botulinum that causes the disease botulism. Botulism is a disease that causes extreme weakness and temporary paralysis of muscles throughout the entire body, and it can be deadly when ingested in large amounts. But don't be afraid; this does not happen with Botox injections. In the purification process this specific group of molecules and proteins gets purified down to microscopic and controlled quantities. Then these microscopic quantities get delivered, through injection, only to the targeted muscle for just the right result that we're looking for.

Neuromodulators work by blocking the signal from the nerve to the muscle. Nerve endings normally trigger muscle movement through a neurotransmitter called acetylcholine. But Botox blocks the release of acetylcholine, so the muscle never gets the signal to contract down. It's like having your electricity shut off because a wire gets cut, except there is no harm to the muscle or the nerve during this blocking process, and the effect wears off after about 3-6 months.

What is it Used For?

Botox has been described and written up for nearly 100 different uses throughout the body. It helps medically for people who have muscle contractures, spasmodic bladders, and migraine headaches. It helps with a variety of skin conditions including hyperhidrosis (too much sweating), Raynaud's disease (vasoconstriction of the fingers), and others. It's even been used to help people with plantar fasciitis of the feet.

On the face we use Botox for the cosmetic benefit of decreasing dynamic lines and wrinkles. As mentioned before, these wrinkles get deeper and deeper with age and can become very prominent. They are a significant sign of aging. Botox can completely reverse them. That's right, it can eliminate these wrinkles. The temporary loss of movement allows the skin to relax and the indented areas of creases and furrows can eventually relax and come out as well. Sometimes these are treated in combination with topical treatments and/or lasers to further improve these areas.

Typical areas treated on the face include the following:

- Glabella ("11 lines") - FDA approved
- Forehead lines - FDA approved
- Lateral canthal lines (crow's feet) - FDA approved
- Nasal lines (bunny lines)
- Excessive gingival display (gummy smile)
- Lip lines (smoker's lines)
- Oral commissure lines (frown lines)

Less well-known areas on the face that can be treated

- Masseter muscles - Botox can treat symptoms associated with temporal-mandibular disorders (aka TMJ or TMD). It can relax hard-clenching masseter muscles and significantly improve the pain, discomfort, teeth grinding, and even headaches that go along with this. There is also a cosmetic improvement when the lower face has become too full from the thickened masseter muscles.

- Temporalis muscles - These muscles can grow out of proportion to the rest of the face, and make it look out of proportion as well. Gum chewing doesn't help. We can inject these areas with Botox and restore balance. This can also help with tension headaches.

- Parotid Gland - As we age, the parotid gland can grow and get far too big. It lies right under the skin just in front of the ear at the jawline. Serial injections of Botox in this area can significantly shrink the size of the parotid gland, but not interfere with overall saliva production.

Vanity vs. Confidence

Every now and then I get a patient who wants to get Botox but feels conflicted. They'll say something like, "I really want to get Botox, but I don't want to be vain." Sometimes these patients will have a strong religious background, and sometimes they will not. Being a religious person myself, I have tried to really understand where these people are coming from. I think it's rooted in the origins of Botox and the misconceived stigma that developed. When Botox first came out in the early 2000s, it was the only real injectable treatment for cosmetic purposes. Unfortunately, it was lumped in with other cosmetic procedures, which at the time were only the big surgical procedures.

Consequently, many people came to regard Botox as similar to cosmetic plastic surgery. While they have some similarities (both help to improve your appearance), they are in VERY different categories. Botox is a simple, quick, minimally-invasive procedure that improves the appearance of skin on your face. It helps to restore sun-damaged skin. With that definition, it's not very different from getting braces on your teeth, or tattoo makeup on your eyebrows or lips (which actually last much longer than Botox).

What I like to focus on is the added self-confidence that Botox can give you. After your Botox injections, you look younger with fewer lines and wrinkles. You feel more confident in your own skin. Maybe you feel more comfortable going out in public. Maybe you're more willing to go out without makeup, which opens up more opportunities for you. You may find yourself saying "yes" to more social opportunities. It's amazing how many more experiences you can have when you're not worrying so much about getting ready and trying to cover-up or hide things. With a little extra confidence, you can greatly increase the number of positive experiences you have.

Botox Can Make You Happier

Botox injections can also lead to higher levels of objective happiness. Yes, you read that right: higher levels of happiness. Some interesting research has also shown that it can treat depression. There are different theories as to how this works, but it's clear that it's more than just the improved cosmetic results. There's something deeper going on. The leading theory is something called the "Facial Feedback Hypothesis." This theory states that there's a feedback loop with facial expressions and emotions. Not only do your emotions affect your facial expressions, but your facial expressions can also influence your emotions.

Have you ever forced yourself to smile when you didn't feel like smiling? What happened? Likely you started to feel a little happier after a few minutes and the smile started to become more genuine. (Try it and see what happens.) This was studied with an ingenious experiment. Test subjects were given a pencil to hold between their teeth forcing them to smile. After a few minutes they removed the pencil and filled out a survey. These test subjects scored significantly happier than the control group who did not do the pencil maneuver. Botox does the same thing, but in reverse. It blocks some of the main muscle groups in the central forehead (glabella) that are associated with negative emotions. The scowling and frowning associated with emotions like anger, disgust, rage, annoyance, and concern are just not there. The muscles are there, but you just can't make the faces like you used to. Botox gives you a 3-6 month break from feeling the full weight of your negative emotions. This tends to make you happier

Chapter 6

Volume Loss and Dermal Fillers

Why Does My Skin Start Sagging?

One of the cruel tricks of nature is to give us beautiful, attractive, and healthy skin in our youth and then slowly take it away as we age. We discussed previously about the aging that happens from sun exposure. But sun exposure isn't the only force working against you. There's also the continual force of gravity pulling you down. In your youth, your skin was strong and healthy and easily resisted this force. But now that your skin is older and weakened by the sun, it's harder to resist this pernicious downward pull. Add to that the nightly pillow-pressure of sleeping on your face, a little weight gain and/or loss through the years, and poof: Suddenly you're starting to look more and more like your mother.

This, of course, is a gradual process. But what's interesting is that you will likely go years without noticing, and then suddenly--boom. There it is, in every mirror, selfie, and FaceTime call. It seems like it happens overnight. Your perky cheeks, which used to rest high near your eyes, are suddenly sagging down near your jawline. The lines from your nose to your mouth (known as the nasolabial fold or parenthesis lines) are deep and grooved. There's a hollow underneath the corner of your mouth that creates "marionette lines." Your temples may look hollowed out like someone who hasn't had enough to eat. Your undereyes (aka tear troughs) become more prominent with dark circles and bulging fat pads. You start to think, "What's happening to me?"

Do I Need a Face Lift?

It used to be that the only option for these age-related changes was a face-lift. If you wanted an improvement, you had to go under the knife. Certainly, this is still a good option for some people, but in my opinion it's very few. I believe that 80-90% of people who think they need a facelift don't need one. In fact, they should not get one. Facelifts can be risky with complications from cutting (blood vessels or nerves get cut). And don't forget the risks associated with going under general anesthesia. And frankly, the results sometimes don't look great. In fact, they can look BAD. If the skin is pulled too tightly it does not look natural. And remember, it's permanent. Add to this the fact that sometimes the suture line doesn't heal well and you may be walking around for the rest of your life with a very noticeable scar around your ear that you have to explain to everyone who asks about it.

No, a facelift is not the best answer for most people. What's the better answer? Dermal fillers. That's right--volumizing injections from dermal fillers. These, when done well, are superior to a face lift in nearly every way. The results look better and more natural, it's safer with fewer complications, and it's cheaper. There's no cutting, no suture line, and no general anesthesia. Only a few pokes with a needle and you can leave the office and go straight to lunch at your favorite Italian restaurant with your friends.

Thinning Out of Deeper Structures

One way that dermal filler does its work is by restoring the volume lost in the deeper structures of the skin. There are deep fat pads and bones of the face that are foundational for structure and personality. They give your face its characteristic look. They contribute to a youthful appearance and natural beauty. Over time the deeper fat pads start to shrink and resorb. They get smaller and smaller until there's almost nothing there. At the same time, the superficial fat compartments may enlarge, especially if you gain any weight. Skeletal structures also start to shrink and get smaller. The net effect is less fullness at the deeper layers and extra fullness and fat superficially. Gravity, smoking, and sun exposure can accelerate this process. Restoring volume to these deeper areas is incredibly important, and filler injections are the perfect thing to do it.

Upper Face

Filler in the upper face is almost always the best place to start. This is where a lot of those deeper fat pads are, and they need more volume. This can also help to lift and restore the skin on the lower face which may have started to sag. The temples and cheeks are the main areas we look at in the upper face. The filler gets placed on bone, and depending on the filler that's used, it can last for up to two years or more. This can also help to correct the "peanut" look of the upper face. This happens when your temples get hollow, and your zygomatic cheek bone starts to look a little too sharp, with not as soft of a contour. This may not be something you notice as much in the mirror because it's not front and center of your face. But when it's corrected, your brain will notice, and it gives you an overall more youthful and beautiful look.

Lower Face

The lower face can be more challenging. There's a lot of movement in the lower face and it gets more sun exposure. It also feels more of the downstream effects of gravity than the upper face, as this is where things start to sag and collect.

"Smoker's Lines" are particularly common and challenging. If you're over 50 you're very likely starting to notice some lines when you pucker your mouth. These are generally most prominent above the upper lip and are known as "smoker's lines" or "barcode lines." I've also heard it described as "Queen Elizabeth Syndrome." Many people get these and indignantly say, "But I've never smoked in my life!" Unfortunately, these are just lines that form as we age and continue to get deeper and deeper unless you do something about them. Men don't get these nearly as much because they have thicker and more abundant hair follicles in this region, which helps their skin to maintain its thickness and integrity. Smoker's Lines generally require a combination approach with laser first, followed by filler. The "big picture view" is very important here. You definitely want to work with someone experienced, with a long-term view in mind. You also want them to be very good at filler to take care of this problem for you.

Another problematic area of the lower face is the marionette zone (area under the lower lip), which can be a dead giveaway to your age. This area slowly loses volume over time and requires constant attention and maintenance. Jowls along the jawline slowly accumulate and destroy your nice tight jawline (along with your confidence). These can be treated with a combination approach of filler along the jawline/chin, Kybella, and Botox of the masseters.

And of course, don't forget about the nasolabial folds between the nose and the lips. These get deeper and deeper over time and are very noticeable since they're front and center in the mirror. It's great to treat these, but you must be careful to not have them overfilled. Even babies have these lines, and without them we start to look a bit simian or ape-like. And you don't want that.

What are the Different Fillers?

Currently in the US there are four companies with FDA approved dermal fillers. Allergan owns the fillers named Juvederm, Voluma, Volbella, and Vollure. Galderma is the company that owns the fillers named Restylane-L, Restylane Lyft (formerly Perlane), Restylane Silk, Refyne, Defyne, and Restylane Kysse. Merz is the company that owns the fillers named Belotero and Radiesse. The newest line of fillers is called Teoxane with the RHA line (RHA 2, RHA 3, and RHA 4). These are fillers that have been available in Europe and Canada for many years and have just recently been approved in the US.

There are many other companies and fillers in the approval pipelines that will be available within the coming years. As you can see, there are many different fillers that can do many different things. They all have a different "personality" as well. Some are firmer and stronger and able to lift the tissue from deeper planes of the face.

Some are lighter and have more ability to spread, and these are more suited for finer and more superficial tissue of the skin. Whatever project you choose to have done, it is very important to pick the right filler (and the right injector) for the job.

Expert vs. Amateur Injectors

Injection technique is very important when it comes to fillers. There are many different techniques and many different injectors, and they are not all created equal. It's sort of like comparing different restaurants. A 3-star restaurant and a 5-star restaurant have access to the same ingredients and same tools. But the 5-star restaurant has a chef with extensive training who has developed incredible experience over time. And this shows in the combinations, decisions, and techniques that seem effortless to everyone else. The final product far exceeds that of the 3-star restaurant.

There are many nuances that go into this discussion, and it's a very important discussion. You want the best of the best when someone is injecting your face. And there are a lot of injectors out there with minimal levels of training. From MDs at the top of the spectrum down to NPs, PAs, RNs, and even medical assistants are sometimes injecting (a lot of this depends on state regulations). It's true that many of these injectors become very good at what they do. But some don't. I have had to fix the work of other injectors many times, and coach them through what to do when they have a complication. As an MD, I will admit that I have a bias in this area. But it's because I know that no other group of healthcare providers is required to go through as much of a rigorous training process. Even the best and brightest of mid-level and lower-level providers have gaps (sometimes big gaps) in their knowledge base, simply because it wasn't part of their training curriculum.

*Disclaimer: Some of the best injectors I've ever seen are mid-levels (even 1-2 nurses). These always tend to be at high-quality medical practices and are supervised by specialty-appropriate physicians (dermatology, plastic surgery, ENT).

One way to separate expert from amateur injectors is to ask for before/after photos. Experts who have been doing this for a long time will have a large bank of before/after photos to choose from. Another way is if they use cannula. Cannula is a device that is like a long hollow straw. It is blunt on the end and is firm but allows for bending when necessary. It also allows for only one puncture of the skin, rather than multiple (as with needles). It takes time and practice to become proficient with cannula. But this reduces the risks of bruising, swelling, and arterial occlusion. While this is not universal (many amazing injectors don't use cannula), it can be a very helpful discussion point. In general, someone who uses a lot of cannulas generally has an appropriate understanding of facial anatomy and respect for potential adverse effects. They have also demonstrated that they have put in the necessary training time to learn these advanced techniques.

Another way to differentiate can be through pricing. Generally, the higher quality injectors will have a large following and will be harder to get in to see. They will not do too many aggressive pricing deals. I would recommend avoiding a practice that uses Groupon to attract new patients. You generally get what you pay for and your facial injections are not something you want to skimp on to save a few dollars.

My Awesome Mom

My awesome mother is now in her 60s, but you'd never know it to spend time with her. She's a lot of fun and makes everyone around her feel younger. A few years ago, she lost some weight, which was awesome for her. The only problem was that it left a bit of loose and sagging skin around her neck and jawline. As I mentioned before, most people who say "I need a facelift" don't really need one. But Mom was probably in the 10-20% of people who say that, and they actually need one. But she was just never going to get a facelift, mostly due to the fear of going under anesthesia for a big surgical procedure. Her only option, then, was injectables and lasers.

I worked on her for about three years whenever she came into town. I felt like we were making very slow progress. She still had a lot of sagging skin, and things just weren't taking off the way I had hoped. Then, at the three-year mark, we got a little more aggressive with the fillers and suddenly--boom! It all came together. Her face, neck, and jawline looked tighter and proportional. Her features looked natural and younger. She now looks great and calls me frequently to say, "I got another compliment today!" She has more spring in her step, and now her outward age more closely resembles her inward age.

Summary for Fillers

- Fillers are an incredible advancement in anti-aging.

- They can prevent the need for a face lift.

- Upper-face and lower-face are very nuanced and require unique approaches.

- There are many fillers out there, with more coming down the pipeline.

- There are many different injectors out there, with a wide variety of cost and quality.

- You want to find an expert injector with an in-depth knowledge of the skin. Don't shop by price.

Chapter 7

Pigment Problems

Jennifer Had Bad Melasma

Jennifer was an awesome patient who eventually became a good friend (as happens with many of my patients). She had a history of bad melasma for many years (more on what this is later). It really affected her confidence, and she didn't feel comfortable going out in public without makeup. She worked as a hairdresser and looking her best was important to her. She was very discouraged about this problem and wanted her skin to look like it used to. She had tried multiple methods to improve this, but nothing seemed to work. In fact, some things seemed to make it worse. When she first came to see me, I started her on some gentle topicals and a gentle laser called Clear & Brilliant. She did two treatments, then was unable to come back for a few months. During that time, the world initiated a big shut down due to the COVID-19 pandemic. She started wearing a mask daily at work, and this made her melasma noticeably worse.

Then we started her on an aggressive topical regimen for three months and combined it with a few moderate chemical peels. There was significant improvement after two weeks on topicals only. But Jennifer hadn't really noticed the improvement yet. This happens for two reasons: 1) You're often quite red and peeling in these first few weeks. 2) When things improve slowly over time it can be hard to remember what it used to look like. So we pulled up her before/after photos and showed her the stark difference. She started crying when she saw the photos. She was so happy to see that her skin and her appearance were returning to how they used to look. She felt like she was getting her old self back and her confidence was coming with it.

What is Dyspigmentation?

Dyspigmentation is a term that basically means you have discoloration from too much pigment that shouldn't be there. The melanocytes are the pigment producing cells in the skin, and they live in the lowest layer of the epidermis. There is normally one melanocyte for every ten basal cells in that layer. The melanocytes have long dendritic arms that connect them to up to 30 regular skin cells (keratinocytes). When you see dark spots on the skin, they can either be from extra accumulation of melanocytes in that area (moles) or extra accumulation of pigment that is produced in those areas.

There are many different forms of dyspigmentation and most of them are caused by (or worsened by) the sun. All skin types can develop dyspigmentation, but it is generally most pronounced in darker skin types. It can be a local spot or two, or it can be a widespread distribution of the face, neck, and chest. It can be hard to point to one clear spot that is an obvious "lesion," rather the entire background is problematic. The following are some of the most common forms of dyspigmentation and pigmented lesions. We'll discuss some of these in more depth.

1. Sunspots
2. Seborrheic Keratosis (SKs)
3. Moles
4. Poikiloderma
5. Melasma

Quick Overview of Common Pigmented Skin Lesions

- Sunspots - The technical term is solar lentigo, and an alternative (and older term) is "liver spot." These are superficial collections of pigment. There is no increase in actual melanocytes, just the pigment production. They are directly related to sun exposure. They are benign, but very noticeable. They are generally very treatable.

- Seborrheic Keratosis – This is also called a "senile wart" (which is a terrible name in my opinion). These are not sun related, just an overgrowth of skin cells that does not fall off effectively. It's basically just a group of cells stuck to the skin's surface. These happen to almost everyone as we age. Some people call them "age spots," but I prefer the more friendly version of "wisdom spots." They are raised and often rough and scaly, sometimes with a shiny appearance. Some people can get a lot of these, especially on the face, scalp, neck, chest, and back. These are very treatable.

- Melasma - This is also known as "chloasma" or "pregnancy mask." It is wide-spread pigment that is blotchy and ill-defined. It behaves in unpredictable ways and randomly gets worse and darker. It is definitely related to sun exposure and heat, but also has a hormonal component as well. It can flare during menstrual cycles or pregnancy. It can be hard to treat, and sometimes gets worse with treatments, especially heat-producing treatments (like certain lasers). If treated correctly, this can be significantly improved. Complete cure is rare as this tends to continue to flare with future triggers. But we can manage it over time.

- Moles - These come in all shapes and sizes and can be anywhere on the body. Some general rules about moles is that over time they start to lose their pigment and become more raised. You also don't want to see any new moles after the age of about 50. If so, we worry about melanoma (more on this later).

- Poikiloderma - This is widespread blotchy discoloration of areas that are exposed to the sun. The face, neck, and scalp areas are most commonly affected. There is generally a mix of red and brown discoloration that becomes blotchy and poorly defined. There are generally other signs of chronic sun exposure present as well (sunspots, growths, telangiectasis, skin atrophy and wrinkles).

- Freckles - These are superficial collections of pigment. They are harmless and contribute to a person's "signature look." These can be removed or decreased in appearance, but I am often hesitant to do so, as these are often a part of you and your personality.

What About Melanoma?

This is a big one and deserves some attention. Whenever there's a pigmented lesion that you're worried about, you should get it looked at by a dermatologist. Often, it will be one of the benign lesions mentioned above. But we never want to miss a possible melanoma. These are sneaky skin cancers that can look like a lot of different things, but most commonly they just look like an abnormal mole. They can behave in very strange and unpredictable ways. They can also become very serious and very deadly. They are much more dangerous than the other, more common forms of skin cancer. They deserve to be respected and evaluated. There are two main frameworks you can use when checking your skin for possible melanoma: ABCDE and "The Ugly Duckling."

ABCDE stands for Asymmetry, Border irregularity, Color that is non-uniform, Diameter larger than 5 cm, and Evolving over time. It's important to remember that benign moles can break some (or all) of these rules. And there are also melanomas that don't break any of them. But it's a good framework to start with.

"The Ugly Duckling" rule helps in situations where you have moles that don't follow the rules. Most people have a signature pattern of moles. They may or may not follow the ABCDE framework. For example, there are many people that have a lot of moles with an irregular border. But they all have the same signature appearance. They may break the same rules in the same ways. But if you see one that breaks a different rule, or just looks different from the rest, then this one is the "ugly duckling" and deserves to be biopsied for a closer look.

Obviously, this is a very complex topic and a very important one. This is why you really need to see a dermatologist if you have any concerns about pigmented lesions at all. It's my opinion that anyone and everyone should have a yearly skin check. But if you're over 50 or if you have fair skin, then it's even more important.

Pigment Controllers

Pigment controllers (aka bleaching agents) were discussed in a previous chapter about topical products. These are important for many different skin conditions and treatment plans. And they are essential for pigment-related conditions. Most of them utilize a medication called hydroquinone as the active ingredient. This is a prescription medication and warrants an important discussion. Hydroquinones work by blocking the pigment production pathway from tyrosine to melanin. This is reversible and only works if you're consistently using the hydroquinone. There are some side effects to be aware of also, mostly in the skin irritation category. We generally recommend that people don't use hydroquinone for too long without taking a little break. My general rule is three months on, and three months off. There are also other "non-hydroquinone" products that don't have as many potential side effects, but also don't seem to work quite as well.

Lasers

There are many lasers that can help with pigment problems as well. This is a topic that must be dealt with very carefully, though. Sometimes lasers can make pigment problems worse. Patients with darker skin types and patients with certain conditions (like melasma) are at a higher risk for this to happen. If you're in one of these categories that doesn't always mean that you can't have any lasers though. More often than not, you can. We just need to be very careful about how and when we use lasers in the process.

A Word of Caution About IPL

IPL (Intense Pulsed Light) has become a very popular "laser" device for improving pigment on the skin (technically it's not a laser since it uses all wavelengths of light above a certain wavelength filter). It is commonly operated at med spas and medical offices by estheticians and laser technicians. You and the laser technician can easily develop a sense of safety and security from this device because it nearly always does a good job safely. However, in darker skin types you must be very careful as you can easily get a burn from this laser which leads to post-inflammatory hyperpigmentation. And a very important point is that this most often happens after you've had a recent tan-- either from a vacation, laying out, tanning bed, or just being outside gardening. Any form of tan makes IPL treatments much riskier.

Summary for Pigment Problems

1. Pigment problems are very common and varied
2. First you need the right diagnosis
3. Only then can you select the right treatment option
4. Virtually all pigment problems can be treated
5. Some can be completely removed (sun spopts, SKs, moles)
6. Some require effort over time (melisma and poikiloderma)
7. If you're ever worried about melanoma then have it looked at by a board-certified Dermatologist

Chapter 8

Skin Growths

Believe it or not, growths on the face can often be overlooked. When we're analyzing for pigment and volume loss, sometimes little growths can take a back seat, but not always. Sometimes people will notice and fixate on these little growths and go crazy about them. I don't want you to get to that point. It's much better (and easier) to remove growths when they're small. Most growths can be categorized as "malignant" (skin cancers), "pre-malignant" (actinic keratosis), and "benign" (everything else). We'll discuss each category with each unique approach and nuances. Many of them are either caused by, or worsened by the sun. Removing these growths is almost always the best approach. You may have a keen attachment to one or two of these growths. Maybe you have a beauty mark that gives you your signature look. But in my experience, most people are much happier with their face and their skin when these growths are removed.

Malignant Growths

The most common form of skin cancer is basal cell carcinoma (BCC), followed closely by squamous cell carcinoma (SCC). These are followed somewhat distantly by melanoma, which we've already covered. There are different subtypes of each of these, but I'll tell you some of the most important things to look for. There are also other skin cancers that can occur, but they are quite rare. We'll focus on the most common features of the most common lesions.

- BCC - Arises from the basal layer of the epidermis. It often has a pearly/shiny appearance. It can bleed easily and cause frequent scabs. It can also be painful to the touch. BCC is sun-related, so look at sun-exposed areas.

- SCC - Arises from higher layers of the epidermis and has a rougher/scaly appearance and texture. It can even have a "skin horn" coming out of it, which is made of keratin and can look somewhat like a thick fingernail. It often has a red appearance that goes along with the scale. These can also ulcerate and scab. They can be sensitive to the touch and are sun-related, so look at sun-exposed areas.

Pre-Malignant Growths

If you've had liquid nitrogen sprayed on your face or arms at your doctor's office, then you've probably had a pre-malignant growth or "pre-cancer." The technical name for these is actinic keratosis (AK), and they are very common. They are caused by sun damage over time, and anywhere from 1% to 10% of them will eventually become a full-blown skin cancer-- always a squamous cell carcinoma (SCC). Most of them will just go away on their own or stay there and do nothing. But given this malignant potential, we like to get rid of them so they never get the chance to turn bad.

There are many ways to remove these, but freezing them with liquid nitrogen is probably the easiest and most common way. If you are getting many of these frozen off at each dermatology visit, then it might be time to consider a more widespread "field therapy" to tackle all of them at once. I have seen patients with hundreds of these on the face/scalp/arms and there was no way to treat them all with liquid nitrogen.

Field therapy can be intense treatments, but the results are nothing short of fantastic. You get rid of hundreds (sometimes thousands) of these microscopic pre-cancerous lesions in one fell swoop. There are chemotherapy creams, light-based treatments, and lasers that can all accomplish this. There is some definite recovery time with these treatments, and it can honestly be quite challenging (especially the first time). They each have their pros and cons and warrant a discussion with a dermatologist.

Benign Growths

Your facial skin is full of underlying structures supporting the skin, much more than other areas of the body. Examples are hair follicles, sweat glands and ducts, oil glands and ducts, more nerves, and a lot of blood vessels. The good news is that these structures give your skin its amazing function and personality. The bad news is that any component of these structures can develop its own little benign growth of cells. There are so many kinds of small benign growths on the face that it takes years of studying them under the microscope to be able to discern them all. Most of them look identical to the naked eye--a smooth dome-shaped bump that is flesh-colored. It's nothing fancy or exciting, it's just there. Here's a list of some of the more common ones.

1. Sebaceous hyperplasia - These are overgrown oil glands that appear mostly on the forehead, temples, and cheeks, and mostly in adults who have more oily skin. They are totally benign and annoying.

They can be treated and removed if done carefully and properly. Unfortunately, they tend to come back.

2. Fibrous papules (angiofibroma) - This is a smooth dome-shaped bump that most often occurs on the nose. It's just a collection of fibrous tissue and blood vessels. The only way to get rid of these is to remove them with a shave biopsy or hyfrecation. It's important to distinguish these from basal cell carcinoma (BCC).

3. Intradermal nevus - The natural life of most nevi (moles) is to lose their pigment over time and become more 3-dimensional. On the face this leads to moles that used to have color (maybe one of them was your beauty mark when you were younger), but now they're just flesh-colored bumps. The only way to get rid of these is to cut them out. This needs to be done carefully so that you don't get a big scar.

4. Seborrheic Keratosis – These are very common benign growths, and they don't always look pigmented. Sometimes they are pink or flesh-colored. But they always seem to have that waxy "stuck-on" appearance. These are very treatable, even on the face. They love the forehead, temples, cheeks, and neck (also the back and chest).

5. Skin cyst - There are a few different types of skin cysts. The most common form is called epidermal inclusion cyst. This is where there's an invagination in the skin that dives down deep and becomes closed off at the top. The skin continues to produce material (oils, keratin, dead skin cells) and this becomes a very tight ball under the skin. These will sometimes drain themselves, and some of the contents will come out. But they will just re-form unless they are cut out completely. They can also become inflamed, where they get

really red and big. When this happens, they are very tender and about four times as big as they used to be. When this occurs, we generally try to calm them down with steroid injections. Once they shrink back down, they are much easier to remove.

6. Milia cyst - Milia are tiny little white dots that occur on the superficial facial skin. They are like the world's smallest and most superficial cysts. They can look like little white heads, but they don't pop out. They must be scored at the top with a blade and then expressed properly to pop out.

7. Cherry angioma - This is a benign collection of blood vessels in the very superficial skin. They are bright red and can look like a mini cherry in the skin. These can be treated effectively by laser or hyfrecation.

General Treatment Options

The most important part of finding the right treatment is to first have the right diagnosis. Some lesions will respond well to one form of treatment but not to another. For example, actinic keratosis can be curetted off by scraping, but it's more likely to come back this way, so the better treatment option is freezing it with liquid nitrogen. Still other lesions will not respond to these less-invasive options at all and need to be cut out completely (deep moles, cysts). Matching each lesion with the correct treatment can be nuanced and may require some discussion. In general, these are the different treatment options.

• Retinoid creams - These are generally not great for treating existing benign growth, but sometimes they can prevent new ones, especially superficial things.

- Chemotherapy creams - The most popular of these is called Efudex (5-fluorouricil). It is great for killing a lot of pre-cancerous lesions (AKs) all at once. It takes about three weeks of daily or twice-daily application. Your skin can look bad while all these different cells are dying. I tell people to prepare to look like a pepperoni pizza for two weeks. You definitely want a dermatologist overseeing your care while you do this one. The results are incredible.

- Liquid nitrogen - This option freezes the lesion, killing the skin cells which eventually blister up and peel off. It only works for superficial lesions and not deeper ones. Also, don't pick at the blisters.

- Curettage (scraping) - This is also for superficial lesions. It can be more precise than liquid nitrogen, and useful when considering the cosmetic outcome.

- Hyfrecation - This is a light cautery that burns or desiccates (dries out) the lesion. It can be helpful when added to curettage, or it can be used by itself. When a very fine tip is used it can pierce into the deeper layers and treat the deeper lesions as well as superficial lesions.

- Laser - These can spot treat or field treat different lesions. You can also combine a growth removal treatment with a laser treatment and heal from both at the same time. A strong laser like CO_2 or Erbium ablative can do the same thing that chemotherapy creams do by removing large numbers of actinic keratoses. And they can also rejuvenate and treat all the surrounding skin as well. It's a great two-for-one option.

Importance of Prepping the Skin

Making sure the skin is well prepped before these procedures is very important. You don't want to remove one benign lesion just to trade it for another. As discussed in previous chapters, any time we traumatize the skin it can react by producing too much or too little pigment. If the sun sees the fresh healing skin, it will cause big problems. These usually resolve over time, but it can take a while. It's always better to prep the skin in advance so this doesn't become a problem. The best way to prep the skin is with a retinoid and a hydroquinone. These topical creams were covered in greater depth in Chapter 3.

Conclusion

Hopefully, at this point you agree with me. Your skin is incredibly important and it's under attack. The forces working against you are persistent, misunderstood, and ubiquitous. You need to care for your skin every day so it can continue to take care of you. You need to prepare for the daily onslaught and prevent future damage. And once the damage occurs, you need to work hard to repair and correct it.

Some may say that all this advice is too much. Too many steps. Too much of a hassle. Too much brain power. Too much money. And on and on. I've heard it all. But since you've read this far you probably agree with me. Your skin is an amazing gift. It's beautiful and functional. It deserves to be protected and repaired. People around you may say they just don't care about their skin. That may be what they say, but deep down, they all want skin that is healthy and looks youthful.

Twenty years from now, how do you want your skin to look? Imagine showing up to your 30th or 40th high school reunion with all your old high school friends. Everyone is the same age, and everyone has had a full life so far. Do you want to look like the oldest person in the room? Or do you want to look like the youngest person in the room? If you want to look younger than everyone else in the room, you can do it. Follow the guidance in this book and it will happen. It's worth it.

Don't be afraid to work on yourself. Don't be afraid to help yourself, or even "treat yo self." You deserve it every now and then. Great skin does not mean a big ego or vanity. It means you care about yourself and there is nothing wrong with caring about yourself. You likely care for others every day of your life.

The confidence that comes from youthful and healthy skin is amazing. When you feel like you're defying the aging process, then you start to look as young as you feel. And you deserves to look as young as you feel.

It's also important to pace yourself and be patient. Things happen slowly with your skin, but if you're putting in the effort then the process is working. It's like running a marathon. You must be patient and just keep moving forward. You'll get there.

If you wanted to transform your body from a sedentary sluggard to active athlete, you'd need to put in hard work over a long period of time. And it would take some time--a year or longer. You also wouldn't be able to do it on your own. You'd need a support system and a great personal trainer/coach, someone to teach you what to do, and someone to be accountable to.

The same is true when transforming your skin. It's not something that can be done overnight, and it's not something you can do by yourself. You need the right trainer/coach to help you through the process, someone to teach you what to do and how to do it. You also need someone to be accountable to. You need a great dermatologist.

And when you get amazing results, don't be afraid to share. This knowledge is not readily available. There's so much misinformation out there and so many products that it gets very confusing very fast. Share what you've found with others so they can start transforming their skin, too. It may also give them permission to start caring for their skin (and themselves) as well.

About the Author

Austin Cope, MD, MBA is a board-certified dermatologist, and passionate about skin health. He practices cosmetic and procedural dermatology at Skin Spectrum Dermatology in Tucson, AZ. His training includes:

- Medical School: Texas Tech University HSC (2011-2015)
- Master of Business Administration (MBA): Texas Tech University Rawls College of Business (2011-1013)
- Transitional Year Internship: Tucson Hospitals Medical Education Program (2015-2016)
- Dermatology Residency: University of Utah Hospitals and Clinic (2016-2019)
  - Chief Resident (2018-2019)

He has also received additional procedural training from world-renown dermatologists Kent Remington, MD, based in Calgary, Canada, and Jody Comstock, MD, based in Tucson, AZ. Austin has always been interested in positive psychology and self-confidence. He believes that skin health is deeply connected to overall personal self-confidence and opens up many doors of opportunity. Austin lives with his amazing wife and five spunky children where they have been changing diapers continuously for over 12 years now. They love to read, play soccer and go to the beach (with proper sun protection of course).

For more information about Dr. Cope and Sun-Proofing your skin, go to **sunproofbook.com**

To book an appointment with Dr. Cope call **(520) 797-8885** or visit **skinspectrum.com**

Acknowledgements

There are a lot of people that deserve my sincerest thanks and gratitude.

- First of all I need to thank my amazing wife Laura. She is a truly remarkable woman who has sacrificed so much and dedicated her life to the hardest and most rewarding work there is – raising our children. This book (or anything of importance in my life) wouldn't have happened without her.

- To Tommy, Annie, Henry, Lucy, and Clayton. Our spunky, funny, kind, awesome kids. I couldn't be prouder of you guys. Thanks for giving me motivation to push forward all these years.

- To Ryan Reeves my high school English teacher (and editor of this book). I don't know who's more surprised that I wrote a book, you or me. Thanks for showing me that it's possible to be a nerd and super-cool at the same time.

- To Jody Comstock and the rest of the Skin Spectrum team. Thanks for welcoming me so warmly into the family. There's no better place to work and serve others.

- To my awesome supportive parents, siblings, and grandparents. Thanks for always being there. I have an amazing family.

- To my patients. Thanks for giving me the opportunity to serve and take care of your skin. Your trust and confidence is a great honor.